The *SHE*
Book of Beauty

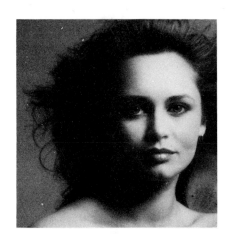

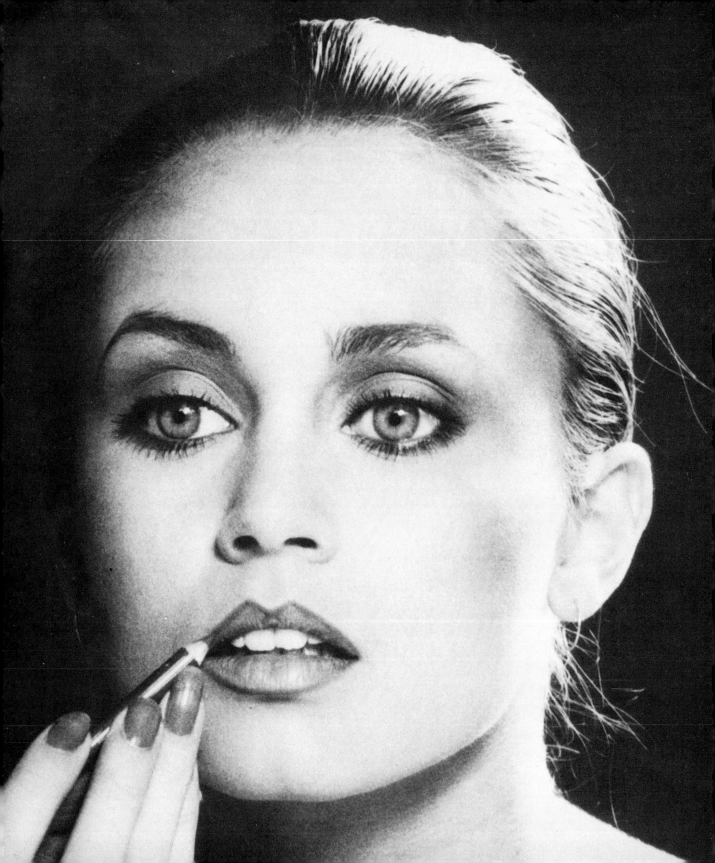

The SHE Book of Beauty

Sally Ann Voak

Book Club Associates
London

This edition published 1979 by Book Club Associates
by arrangement with Arthur Barker Limited

Published in Great Britain by Arthur Barker Limited
91 Clapham High Street, London SW4 7TA

COVER PHOTOGRAPH BY COURTESY OF LANCÔME

Foundation is Maquisatin Miel Doré with creamy blusher Fondants à Joues, Mandarine
Glacée; the slightly shimmering effect is created by using Maquifinish loose powder in
Transparent Nacré. The brow bone is highlighted with Mono Ombres Douces
Champagne d'Or with Pepin d'Or to shade and emphasize the eyes. The Chocolate end
of Le Crayon is used to line the lower lid and Immencils, Lancôme's mascara for sensitive
eyes, is Noir. The lips are outlined and and filled in with Stylo à Lèvres, Cannelle.

Set, printed and bound in Great Britain by
Fakenham Press Limited, Fakenham, Norfolk

Contents

Acknowledgements

The illustrations in this book are reproduced by courtesy of the following:

Almay Hypo-Allergenic Cosmetics: 35, 36
Ambre Solaire: 59
Elizabeth Arden: 55
Bruce Colman Limited: 29
Christian Dior: 61 (photo: Peter Knapp)
Behram Kapadia: 49
Bob Komar: 25
Estée Lauder: 10, 62
Vince Loden: 16, 22, 31, 37, 60, 62, 63, 66, 67, 68, 69, 89, 90, 91, 92, 93 (make-up by Patti
    Burris for Almay, hair by Anestis of Toni and Guy, Davies Street, London W1)
Sandra Lousada: 44
Macdonald Educational Limited: 14
Mercedes-Benz: 82
No. 7 Cosmetics: 52, 53
L'Oréal: 77, 78
SHE: 20
Rosalyn Toohig: 38, 39, 40, 41, 64
Weidenfeld and Nicolson Archive: 27, 30, 47, 58, 70, 72

Note All prices mentioned in this book are correct at the time of publication.

Introduction

The subjects of beauty and vitality are treated seriously and in great depth in *SHE* magazine. Yet the articles I write on looking good and feeling terrific often turn out to be more giggly than gloomy. The reason? To my mind, wit and laughter are essential ingredients in the art of being attractive. You can't look great if you're so serious about beauty care that you lose your sense of proportion. The saddest thing I ever read was the tale of a top beauty who was so hung up on her looks that she plucked out the hairs on her legs one by one to relieve the monotony of thinking about herself!

Frankly that isn't for me or, I hope, my readers. What is? The kind of beauty care I've covered in detail in this book. The kind that isn't sexist (men have much the same beauty problems as women . . . they just aren't conditioned to talk about them so much!); the kind that's based on fact, not meaningless ritual; the kind that takes a cool, often off-beat look at the Body Beautiful; and most important, the kind that boosts your morale without inflating your overdraft.

I hope you'll find it useful and even funny! For more in the same vein (plus fantastic features, fabulous fashion, outrageous puns and great jokes) place a regular monthly order for *SHE*. It's *so* beautifying!

Sally Ann Voak
January 1979

1 Your Health, Your Beauty

Beauty, vitality and good health *must* go together. The current craze for healthy living – jogging, sports, health foods, plenty of sex(!) – is fine, so long as it isn't just a surface idea. You can still feel (and look) ghastly, however many miles you jog before breakfast, if you're suffering from some deeper health problem like acute stress, hormonal imbalance or depression. Unfortunately, both sexes sometimes reach a critical health position before they consult their doctor – and even then, wrong advice or hasty diagnosis can result in disaster. You can't blame doctors for dishing out tranquillizers if you don't take the time and trouble to monitor your own body and give them all the relevant facts.

However, not all health-related beauty problems are so serious that they need professional attention. Some, like the 'curse', just need common sense. Here's a list of common problems, with ideas on treatment.

Pre-menstrual and menstrual problems Just before the 'curse' most women experience slight pre-menstrual tension and fluid retention . . . some get more than their fair share of both horrors. Most of us feel puffed up (the scales can record between 2 lbs and 7 lbs of extra weight to prove that fluid retention is *not* a feminine myth) and decidedly tetchy. If you're on the Pill, the tetchiness may be less marked, the fluid retention more so. Plan a low-salt diet (but don't be disappointed if you're slimming frantically and there is no weight-loss at all), keep cool and treat yourself to a beauty treat like a hair-do, massage, professional make-up session or facial during that difficult week. There's nothing like a bit of luxurious self-indulgence to make you feel less bitchy. If the bitchiness gets out of control, see your doctor. Thanks to the pioneering work of pre-menstrual tension specialist Dr Katharina Dalton, GPs now recognize this as a hormonal syndrome, not just an inconvenience which women are doomed to suffer. Vitamin B6 and a hormone called dydrogesterone are often prescribed for pre-menstrual tension sufferers.

If your period is very heavy (a common problem with women who now have a coil contraceptive), you must make sure you take in extra iron during and after your period, otherwise you'll feel run down, pale and listless – and you'll look awful. You can buy an iron supplement from the chemist, or better still you can eat liver, kidneys, green vegetables and drink a pint of stout every day. Be brilliant, witty, artistic, but don't try to be too physical. Two baths a day will make you feel fresher and livelier; so will a couple of early nights with a good book. *Don't* crash diet, fast, or go on the wagon during your period. *Do* eat an orange at every meal (vitamin C helps the body absorb iron), and spoil yourself a little.

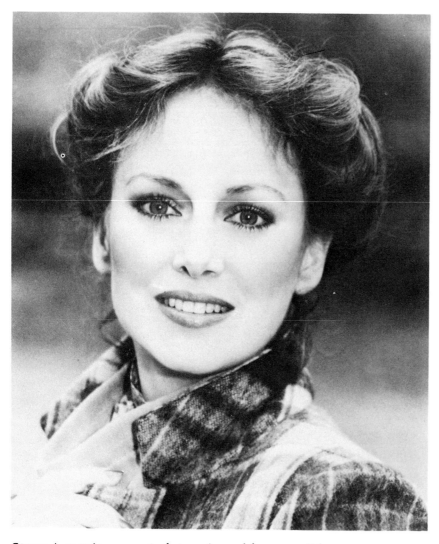

Looking healthy is more than half the battle in looking beautiful.

Stress A certain amount of stress is *good* for you – it keeps you on your mettle, feeling alive, feeling necessary. But in this modern age of hectic lifestyles, relentless pressure and our competitive society, it's quite poss- ible to be over-stretched to the point of sacrificing your health, strength and peace of mind. Hardly a recipe for beauty! Researchers on the subject at Nottingham University's Stress Unit have found that repetitive, boring jobs are more likely to cause stress than demanding, exciting ones and that the combination of several mildly nasty experiences like moving house, changing jobs or having a row with the boss are more likely to cause stress symptoms than one traumatic experience like a death in the family or a divorce.

Here's a list of ten questions to determine your stress-level. More than six 'yeses' and you need to re-assess your life *now*.

1 Do you sleep badly and/or wake up tired?
2 Do you find it impossible to hear people out without interrupting?
3 Do you talk to yourself *often*? (Occasional outbursts don't count!)
4 Do you complain more than once a week that no one understands you?
5 Would you rather go somewhere else than wait in a queue in a shop?
6 Have you suffered any *three* of the following traumatic experiences recently? Change of job, moving house, break-up of a relationship, death in the family, redundancy, demotion, promotion, birth of a child, a holiday (experts say holidays are usually more upsetting than relaxing!), marriage, vasectomy or sterilization operation, any accident or illness.
7 Are you incapable of holding a sheet of paper at arm's length without making it tremble?
8 Do you drink alone more than three times a week?
9 Does a criticism upset you – even a minor one which you know is justified?
10 Have you any nervous habits such as twisting your fingers, pulling your hair, grinding your teeth, biting your nails, chain-smoking?

It's all very well to say 're-assess your life', but it's difficult to put into practice. Sometimes, very simple things can stop you twitching, over-drinking and help smooth out that troubled brow. For instance, selling your car may give you a much easier life – a period of rest and tranquillity while travelling to work each day. Or, just try *not* to do the vital jobs like shopping, going to the cleaners, having your hair cut, taking the dog to the vet all on one busy Friday when work is also frantic. Try saying 'no, sorry' more often to your boss, your kids, your lover (not *too* often!). Martyrs are their own worst enemy, and often not appreciated as much as the selfish types who swan around with unlined faces, perfect teeth (*they* have time for orthodontics) and happy grins. Doctors recommend taking holidays in short, frequent intervals rather than two- or three-week chunks. Or, suggest doing a four-day week with longer hours ... more firms are using this system which encourages employees to take up hobbies like yachting, flying and brass-rubbing which make them more interesting as well as more relaxed people.

Personally, I find that nothing makes me more twitchy than knowing I look a mess. An instant cure for that uptight feeling is a two-hour session at the hairdresser's (I do take work with me – but I don't tell people where I'm going) or painting my nails in bed while sipping a blend of whisky, lemon juice, hot water and honey.

Other instant anti-stress ideas Playing football in the park, a solitary six-length swim, *not* watching TV for a week, reading a magazine which doesn't scream opinions at me, doing a little quiet crochet or knitting, cleaning the car, going for a jog around the block, listening to classical guitar music, sex, a daily top-up of vitamin B6, a day by the sea, gardening, a game of squash, sketching, walking in the rain.

Hormones and the menopause Recently, there has been a lot of publicity about the pros and cons of hormone replacement therapy for menopausal problems such as hot flushes, vaginitis and brittle bones. Medical opinion is divided about the value of the treatment but there is evidence that the combined use of oestrogens and progesterone can be helpful to some women. If you experience severe symptoms of this kind, your doctor (or the organization mentioned in the beauty addresses at the end of this book) can put you in touch with a clinic dealing with menopausal problems.

Beauty problems associated with the menopause include dry, sagging skin, facial hair, pigmentation patches on face, arms and hands, constipation, fatigue. (Cheer up, these problems crop up in teenagers and during the sexy thirties too!) Treat your skin to new, intensive care nourishing creams, especially the neck and upper arm areas which contain fewer sebaceous glands than the facial area and quickly become dry. Gentle, upwards massage after the bath when your skin is warm and relaxed can help. Don't just grin and bear facial hair – pluck out individual hairs with tweezers if there are just a few of them. If you're bristling away, have the hairs removed by electrolysis. *Downy moustaches* can be removed by waxing. *Pigmentation patches* can be disguised with blemish sticks and a covering of liquid foundation topped by a little powder. *Constipation and fatigue* are often caused by the psychological problems associated with the 'change of life' much more than hormonal changes. Avoid taking headache pills, and take extra care with diet: roughage such as bran and raw vegetables can help the constipation problem and extra B and C vitamin foods (citrus fruit, vegetables, wholewheat bread) can cure tiredness.

More than ever, a woman at this stage needs body-toning exercises: embark now on a course of yoga or similar exercises and you'll be surprised how much fitter and more vital you feel. Work, of course, is the great antidote to menopausal, or any other, blues. It's also a great recipe for good health, generally!

2 All About Your Skin

There's about eighteen square feet of skin on your body . . . it's the 'paper bag' that keeps you intact! So, it's an important working bodily organ as well as a source of beauty. If you cut a section through your skin you'd find that it's composed of closely-connected layers. The three main layers are: the epidermis (outer covering), the dermis (which lies just below the epidermis) and the subdermis (below the dermis and a part of the subcutaneous tissue).

The epidermis itself has five distinct layers: the stratum corneum, stratum lucidum, stratum granulosum, stratum spinosum and stratum germinativum. The dermis contains the sebaceous glands which produce sebum (or body oil), sweat glands and hair follicles plus the vital nerve endings. Cosmetics can penetrate only the epidermis, otherwise they are classified as drugs. However, recent research has shown that cosmetics and face creams can create more dramatic changes than was realized a few years ago – but more of that later.

Here's a blow-by-blow account of the function and structure of the five layers of the epidermis:

Stratum corneum (or horny layer) This is the outside covering composed of seven different layers of cells, each one thin and flat. These cells have lost water on the way up from the stratum germinativum; by the time they reach the surface they contain about 15 per cent water, which gives the skin its bloom and soft appearance.

Stratum lucidum (or clear layer) This consists of three separate layers of clear cells. These cells are waiting to journey upwards to the stratum corneum.

Stratum granulosum (or granular layer) Under a microscope you'd see that this layer is only one or two cells thick and has a granular appearance, since each of the cells is filled with little granules.

Stratum spinosum (or spiny layer) This consists of about fifteen layers of cells which have a spiny appearance. Little projections fit together so that one cell hooks up with the next. It's vital to keep these cells hooked up, otherwise your skin would drop off! In fact, at the ripe old age of seventy or so, you start losing the little projections between the cells and your skin starts 'slipping'.

Stratum germinativum (or germinating layer) This is the only cell layer that's actually alive: each cell in this layer divides and journeys upwards through the other four layers to arrive finally on the skin's surface. This constant renewal process takes about seventeen to twenty-three days.

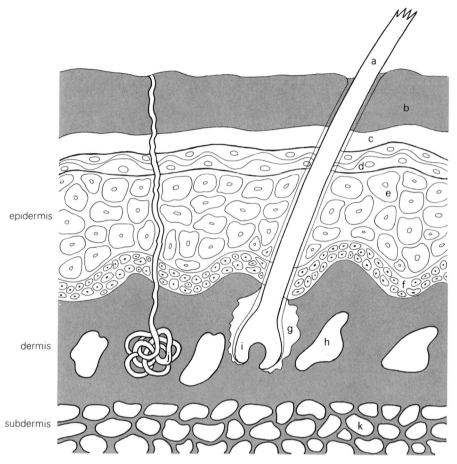

Skin is a highly complicated structure. This diagram shows:

a hair shaft
b stratum corneum
c stratum lucidum
d stratum granulosum
e stratum spinosum
f stratum germinativum
g sebaceous gland
h blood vessels
i papilla
j sweat gland and duct
k fatty tissue

You can see that the top five layers of your skin are very busy – a constantly changing 'procession' of cells rising to the top and undergoing a fascinating conversion process on the way up. What happens is that the cells lose water on the journey, converting their juicy protoplasm to keratin protein. This is the same kind of protein that makes up hair and nails, but in the skin it's much softer, retaining that 15 per cent of water I mentioned earlier, and with a different molecular structure . . . a much weaker 'hooked-together' form than the harder type of keratin.

Meanwhile, down in the dermis, there's a lot going on too. As already mentioned, this layer contains a veritable power-house of working parts from the sebaceous glands to the nerve endings that give your skin its 'feelings'. Here, the sebaceous glands pump sebum into the hair follicles or 'pores' of the skin to produce a protective and softening covering on top of the horny layer. This pumping process is controlled by hormonal factors which, in turn, are influenced by bodily rhythms and developments like puberty, menstruation and the menopause.

How can you keep your skin looking good? First, it's vital to realize that *water* is the main ingredient of a soft, youthful-looking skin. Unfortunately, central heating, the elements and the ageing process all conspire to rob the skin of this vital moisture. There are many creams on the market which help prevent moisture-loss by adding a fine layer of protective oily film over the skin. These 'occlusive' creams can certainly help when you're up against wind, rain and day-to-day skin-drying villains. They also provide a good base for make-up and powder. However, the creams don't soften the skin . . . it's water that does that! A recent development in skin creams on the continent has produced a molecular structure which actually regulates the water-content of the skin, according to the conditions experienced. It's a net-like structure, very sparingly applied, which really helps that water-loss problem. These creams (Vichy's Equalia, for example) are now widely available from chemists here, too.

Can diet help? Doctors are divided about the role diet plays in skin health. However, it's a fact that the skin is made from protein and needs protein to be renewed. If you eat insufficient protein (or incomplete proteins which do not contain all the amino-acids needed to process the protein), your muscles will lose tone, your skin will become muddy-looking and dry, and wrinkles will appear. It's widely assumed that the Western diet is packed with protein, but this is not always the case – you may, for instance, have trimmed your housekeeping budget by cutting down the amount of meat and fish you eat. Remember that there are other good sources of proteins: brewer's yeast, nuts, soya beans, milk, liver, and kidneys. As you get older, you should aim to check that your skin is getting its fair share – at least 100 grams a day. If you are a vegetarian, you need to be extra careful about your protein intake. Other nutrients which, indirectly but diligently, work for the health of your skin are: Vitamin B complex (yeast, wheatgerm, liver, kidneys), Vitamin C (citrus fruits). Baddies are booze (which dilates blood vessels and dehydrates the whole body, including the skin), fried foods and sugary foods.

What about open pores and acne? Pores (which are really hair follicles, see above) are really tiny tunnels through which sweat and sebum are constantly pumped. The sebaceous glands in the dermis are about three to four times as large in the 'T-zone' of the face – across the forehead, down the nose, across the upper lip and on the chin. So, these areas tend to be oilier. No lotion will 'close' pores although some manufacturers claim that their products will do so. In fact, many 'pore tighteners' simply irritate the pores, setting up a swelling reaction which gives a temporary appearance of a smoother skin. However, the pore opening will often take on a 'funnel' appearance where deposits of sebum and debris have gathered around the opening; the funnel is wider at the top, narrower at the bottom. If the face is scrupulously cleaned to remove the debris, the

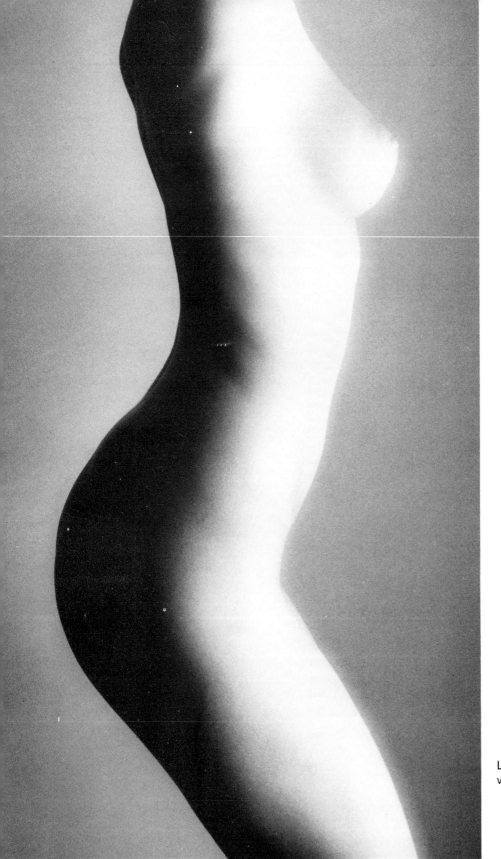

Look after your skin with care and it will feel as good as it looks.

pores will certainly appear much smaller; a good cleanser followed by a skin tonic can help here. Always use a non-greasy make-up on these areas to minimize the amount of grease on the face. If the open pores are pumping out more sebum than they can cope with, then spots and acne can result. The over-activity is triggered off by hormonal activity – the 'baddie' is a male hormone called androgen which is especially active during puberty; this is why puberty is usually the spottiest time of your life. Treatment? Again, doctors are divided about the value of dietary treatment, but I am convinced that acne *is* aggravated by fatty, fried foods – the teenage favourites like hamburgers, chips, sausages, and cakes.

Here is a detailed account of how acne develops:

1 Hormone activity (see above) overstimulates the release of sebum, making the skin too greasy.
2 The flow of sebum eventually plugs the sebaceous gland openings – they just can't cope!
3 The plugged duct stops flowing and a whitehead (milia) becomes visible just under the skin surface.
4 As it becomes exposed to the air, it oxidizes and turns black, becoming a blackhead (comedone).
5 Often, the horny layer of the skin has by then grown over the duct outlet, so the blockage cannot escape. It becomes a red raised bump or pimple. The body's defence system rushes white blood cells to join battle with invading bacteria and pus forms. You're left with a nasty, infectious mess called a pus pimple.

Unfortunately, fiddling with and squeezing pimples usually spreads the infection. Here's a guide to what you *should* do:

1 Wash an oily skin at least three times a day with a mild soap to prevent oil build-up.
2 Don't pick pimples. *Do* extract blackheads with a clean blackhead extractor and washed fingers.
3 Use a light, hypo-allergenic make-up (worrying about pimples can make them worse, so camouflage does help your problem) and loose powder.
4 Shampoo regularly with a mild shampoo and keep hair off your face and back.
5 Watch your diet and step up *roughage* – constipation may mean that toxins have to escape from the body by other means, i.e. through the skin. You have enough problems in that area already.

Seek advice from a dermatologist if the problem is getting out of hand. He will prescribe drying agents, or antibiotics such as tetracycline to help reduce the acid concentrations in the sebum. Or, he may recommend dermabrasion (skin peeling done surgically), or a course of contraceptive pills. The Pill contains oestrogen which tends to control acne; people who are taking it often find their skin improves. The reason why women often have a pimple or two just before their period is that the oestrogen production in the body reaches its lowest ebb at that particular time in the monthly cycle.

Boys with acne usually find that the problem clears up quickly once they pass the difficult puberty years. However, they can take away much of the agony with sensible treatment. There is certainly no need for a teenager to suffer agonies of embarrassment these days. But mums with teenage boys must bully them a little to make sure they do stick to the hygiene rules above and watch their diets!

What's the best treatment for dry skin? If you have dry skin (or even just an excessively dry area on your cheeks), then you could face a wrinkly future! You need extra skin care using the *humectant* type of skin preparation. This differs from the *occlusive* creams described above in that it actually draws moisture from the air to replenish the skin's own depleted moisture supply. It usually penetrates into the stratum corneum, or even deeper into the epidermis, where it deposits the moisture 'plucked from thin air'. The ingredients in these preparations vary, but some manufacturers have managed almost to duplicate the skin's own natural moisturizing factors by using hydrolized proteins, carbohydrate and cow collagen. The advantage of these creams is that they can be worn under make-up and don't give a greasy look to the skin at night. They are, of course, excellent for male dry skins too. If your skin is very dry, you'll also need extra, occlusive-type protection if you go out into very cold weather, wind, or work in a drying atmosphere. Where thread veins are showing in the cheek areas, you should be extra careful with creams and make-up – but these veins can be treated with a form of sclerotherapy which disperses the blood vessels and makes the skin heal up rather like a bruise. (See address list on page 104 for a beauty clinic specializing in this treatment.)

Everyone, even those with oily skins, has a dry neck. The neck area contains fewer sebaceous glands than the face – and therefore needs extra treatment and care. So save some of your special creams and lotions for your neck. The same goes for the eye area; although this area should be treated with great care as the skin is so delicate. Some manufacturers make especially light, easily-absorbed humectants for the eye area; they should be patted lightly on to the skin with the pads of the fingers, not rubbed in. Although they won't prevent wrinkles or whisk them away, they will slow down the wrinkling process and soften already formed wrinkles, making them appear less defined.

Are bags and blemishes treatable? There's a lot you can do to disguise bags and blemishes (see make-up section on page 95), but you should check first whether they can be treated in other ways:

Bags Many women actually cause bags under the eyes by applying too much night cream which becomes trapped under the skin during the night. Try using light cream only, and drink lots of water to help drain fluids out of the system naturally. Make your first drink in the morning a glass of cold mineral water.

Moles Moles can be removed surgically – but you mustn't try to do the job yourself (with wart remover, for instance). Ask your doctor or beautician for advice.

Facial hair Your beard can be plucked out if it's not too obvious (a few hairs, perhaps), or removed permanently with electrolysis (see address list on page 104). This process leaves small pin-prick scabs which heal up quickly.

Freckles and 'liver spots' Freckles are usually very attractive, but if you hate them then the best treatment is to stay out of the sun and use a pale foundation shade. However, 'chloasma' or liver spots may be caused by hormonal activity during pregnancy or by the chemical reaction of the sun on the Pill's essential hormone, progesterone. There are 'whitening' creams on the market for both kinds of pigmentation patches but their effect is rather limited, I'm afraid.

Who gets allergies? Everyone! Most of us are allergic to something or other . . . and all of us are allergic to one thing, the sun – but fortunately the body reacts with first aid in the form of protective melanin pigment cells. Allergic reactions can be triggered off by food, cosmetics, scent, household cleaners, fumes, you name it! Hypo-allergenic cosmetics 'screen out' as many allergens as is practical (which isn't as many as you'd imagine . . . they have to contain preservatives, for example), and some cosmetic companies which don't advertise themselves as 'non-allergic' are also pretty hot on screening out the baddies. French cosmetics, for instance, are closely scrutinized by the health authorities there; even the packaging must be edible. We're not so rigorous in standards here, although legislation is slowly and laboriously being set up to ensure that ingredients are at least listed on the container (which *doesn't* happen at the moment). If you have an allergic reaction to a product the obvious answer is to stop using it. However, it may be difficult to trace the source of the problem, in which case stop using cosmetics for a few days and gradually re-introduce them until you've sorted out the villain. Common allergens are the acetone in nail polish removers, lanolin in cosmetic creams, lead compounds in hair dyes, perfume oils in almost all cosmetics, and sulfonamide resins in nail lacquers.

3 Beauty in Deeper Shades

Just as white skins can't be lumped together under one beauty heading, the many shades of coloured skins can't be treated as one type. Each skin is individual, and potentially beautiful too. But it is a fact that dark-skinned girls do have to try harder to find the right cosmetics and beauty products as they are not yet readily available, despite repeated attempts by manufacturers to launch 'coloured' ranges. Here's a guide to the three main shade-types and how to treat them:

Black skin The rich, dark African skin often has plummy-coloured lights. It's also often quite dry, going flaky and whitish. For that reason, it needs regular lubrication with a good moisturizer and lots of body lotion. Make-up should be very carefully chosen – I recommend the Leichner foundation shades. Powder looks wrong on black skins, but eye make-up is vital – try black kohl pencil around the rim of the lid, plum or brown eye colours and lots of black mascara. Garish blues and greens look wrong – choose subtle colours instead. Soft wand-type lip gloss sticks in chestnut, plum or rose look good on full lips which should be outlined with dark brown pencil.

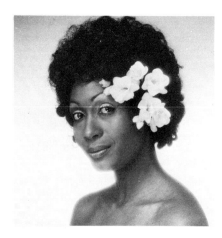

Very dark skin needs only the subtlest of colours.

Coffee skin The paler West Indian colouring can vary from a light brown to deep dark coffee. Rose Laird make a foundation called Tahitian Glow which is very good on the darker coffee colour. Otherwise, the shades for suntanned white skins are often successful on dark skins. Tawny blusher on the cheekbones can help make a very broad face look slightly narrower, plus brown and beige eye shadows and a brown kohl line. *Lots* of mascara suits darker girls but full lips look wrong with bright lipstick. Experiment with soft, subtle colours.

Olive skin This type of Oriental skin colour can look very yellowish and dull in winter although it glows beautifully in summer. Accentuate the glow with a coppery foundation, amber blusher, and golds and browns around the eyes. Rust-coloured lips topped with gloss look pretty too. Essential: brown kohl pencil round the eyes or to add depth and shape to almond eyes.

A great bonus for dark-skinned girls is the fact that coloured skins wrinkle less quickly than white skins – for a start, their owners *aren't* tempted to spend hours baking in the sun.

If you have a difficult skin colour, it's well worth investing in a make-up session at a salon where most manufacturers are represented (see

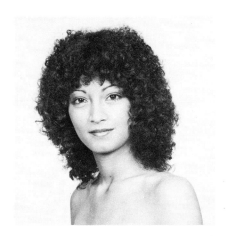

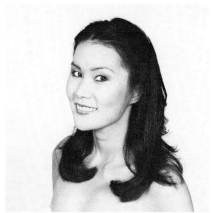

It's worth experimenting with lots of shades of eye shadows and blushers to get the best from a medium brown skin.

If you have Oriental colouring, play up your eyes with browns and mauves.

addresses on page 104). Experts will help you find the perfect colours for your skin – without costly mistakes.

Hair Coloured girls often have dry, difficult hair which is difficult to style. Coconut oil (from chemists everywhere) is an excellent conditioner. You can also give your hair an olive oil treatment: smother hair in warmed olive oil, wrap in a towel and leave for one hour before shampooing. Straightening techniques can be very harmful – the reverse perming process used puts a lot of strain on the hair. It's better to wear your hair in a natural curl or plait or twist it into a pretty style. Have it trimmed regularly to get rid of split ends.

4 Your Looks and Your Love-Life

Psychologically, sex and a loving relationship are tremendous beauty boosters. But what many people don't realize is that sex is *physically* beautifying too! Two Italian dermatologists actually ran a series of tests on women in and out of love and they found that oily and dry skins tend to become normal during a satisfying 'affair', all skins become firmer and smoother, dry dull nails acquire sheen and elasticity, and hair grows glossy and thick. There is also a slight increase in moisture in the skin, which gives a helpful boost to the anti-ageing processes.

Why does it all happen? According to the doctors, the delicious emotional 'high', that feeling of walking on cloud nine, has a stimulating effect on the body's para-sympathetic system and the production of oestrogens in the body . . . the hormones responsible to a great extent for 'feminine' attributes like soft skin. Personally, I feel the psychological

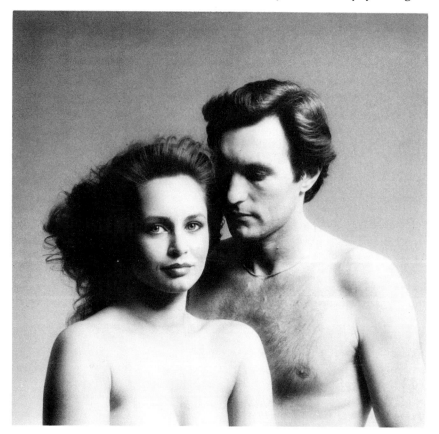

Sex and a loving relationship are terrific beauty boosters.

uplift is even more important than the physical one – when there's a reason to look and feel beautiful, the body is directed by the brain to perk up and look smashing. There's nothing like a new love (or a super old love) to give you a good excuse for washing your hair, putting on a new face, standing up straight and holding your tummy in. Conversely, a broken affair usually means a period of 'going to seed' before you dive into the love scene again after a night of vigorous shampooing! Equally important, there's nothing like *deliberate* concentration on beauty, health and grooming to help you get over a bad patch.

My recipe for mending a broken heart? *Don't* join a car maintenance class – spend the money on a day at a luxury beauty salon instead! If cash is short, splurge on some bath oil, a good shampoo and a delicious bottle of wine. All three are great investments.

Sexual intercourse itself is a rapid beauty treatment which does wonders for your looks; this time the effects are more physical and emotional although, obviously, happiness helps! Before intercourse, pupils dilate and eyes shine (they stay shiny right through), posture improves and breasts increase in size. The pectoral muscles which hold up the breasts 'twitch' slightly giving an isometric exercise which is quite involuntary but extremely beneficial for perking up droopy breasts. Then, the side walls of your nose expand slightly, making your nostrils wider which, in turn, makes you breathe much deeper, taking in oxygen which is vital for beauty functions like cell renewal, hair and nail growth. Since most of us breathe badly, in a very shallow fashion most of the time, this heady sensation produces dizziness and lightheadedness (passion?). There is now a body temperature increase of two or three degrees, and then blood pressure is raised slightly and circulation is stepped up. All three things make you feel alive and glowing and are good for you – unless you are a fatty or have heart trouble (although heart specialists are now actually *recommending* sex and light exercise for post heart-attack patients). There is also a sudden increase in the secretion of the hormones oestrogen, progesterone, androgen and testosterone plus a super boost in muscular exercise in the thighs, tummy and buttock regions. As these areas don't get much exercise normally, daily sex (if you can manage it) is terrific just before you go on holiday and reveal almost all in a teeny bikini.

However, sex is overrated as a slimming pastime, if you're the type who likes to eat afterwards. It does 'burn off' around 200 calories and, according to psychologists, a warm loving relationship can help reduce your craving for 'comfort' foods like sugar, sweets and booze, which are all notoriously high in calories, and low in nutritional value. So, if you can steer yourself away from late-night snacks, sex will certainly have nutritional benefits.

As an anti-stress treatment, intercourse is second to none. Stress contributes to nasties like wrinkles, headaches, premature baldness and grey hair, bad breath, dandruff, and acne, so anything that helps you relax is obviously a good beauty treatment. Sleep *after* sex is usually the deep, refreshing kind, not the kind that makes you feel more tired in the morning than you were at night. So sex is just what the doctor ordered for insomnia too.

Bedtime exercises If you want to improve your sexual performance (and therefore your looks – see above), you need a supple, relaxed body. Try these exercises in bed; they are also good if you're temporarily without a sex partner and feel like limbering up.

Curl-ups Lie on your right side, and curl up into a ball hugging your knees. Now stretch out, arms above your head, toes pointed. Curl up again, roll over to your left side, stretch and repeat five times. Good for your back, tummy and posture.

Thigh twists Sit back against the pillows supporting your weight on your hands. Now open your legs, turn the toes of your left foot inwards, raise left leg off the bed slightly and cross it over your right leg as high as you can go. Swing it back to starting position, then repeat with right leg. Repeat whole exercise five times for strong thigh muscles and taut tummy muscles.

Back kicks Roll over and lie on your tummy, hands by your sides, head on one side flat on the bed (no pillows this time). Now raise left leg as high as possible, cross over right leg, and lower so that your big toe touches the sheet. Raise again, cross back over right leg and lower. Repeat with right leg. Repeat whole exercise five times.

Bedtime beauty Don't go to bed in curlers or saggy winceyette pyjamas if you want to be loved – I'm talking to men as well as girls. A top hair-dresser tells me he actually advises his male clients to wear a hairnet in bed to protect their blown-dry coiffeurs from getting rubbed up the wrong way at night . . . sad. Here's advice for both sexes:

For her Twenty-four-hour mascara may look good in bed in the TV commercials, but it's very bad for your eyelashes. Instead, wear a little kohl pencil above lower lashes, brush brows well and use a little lip-gloss and blusher. Night creams should be applied well in advance so they sink in before bedtime. *Essential*: lashings of perfume, clean feet, sparkling teeth (remove red wine stains from lips too), and brushed hair.

For him Soften hands with hand cream and clean nails, brush your hair (forget the hairnet), apply after-shave or toilet water, clean your teeth thoroughly to remove beer fumes from your breath. *Essential*: undress carefully so you're *not* observed wearing just your socks. Even the most divine-looking guy could find his authority undermined in that situation.

For both Boredom is death to even the cosiest relationship. So, try seeing each other in a different light – literally. Change your room around, swap lighting, change your practical non-iron brown sheets for sexy satin ones. You'll both look very different, and feel it too.

5 Thought for Food

In the next few years, nutrition will be the most talked-about science. For, at long last, doctors are getting together with nutritionists and biochemists to explore fully the relationship between what we eat and what we are. They're coming up with dietary treatments for physical and mental diseases which would have been scorned ten years ago. As a confirmed 'beauty food' addict, I believe that diet really does make a difference to the way you look, feel and act. So the first essential in making the most of your looks is to watch your diet very carefully indeed. You may not be able to change the shape of your nose, the colour of your hair or the size of your feet by eating correctly, but you can make a fantastic difference to the

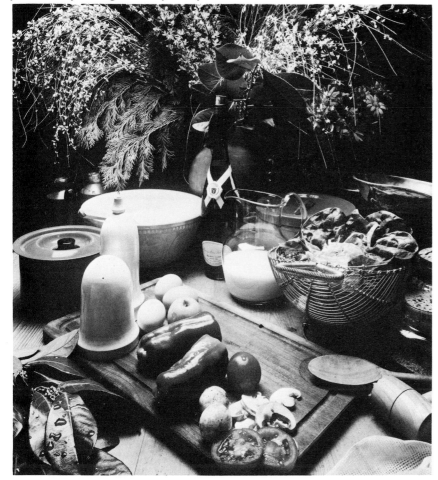

Eating a wide range of fresh foods is one of the most important aspects of feeling and looking your best.

quality of the raw material you were blessed (or cursed!) with.

Here's a guide to the foods you need for each beauty asset:

Shiny hair In order to grow strong and thick, hair needs a regular 'diet' of protein foods (fish, eggs, meat, soya products, lentils). It also needs iron for healthy blood circulation to the follicle and hair root: vitamin B2 (in yeast, wheatgerm, liver, kidneys, wholewheat bread, lean meat), magnesium (green salads, green vegetables, nuts, whole grains), phosphorus (milk, cheese, egg yolk, yeast, wholemeal bread). Of these nutrients, the B complex is perhaps the most interesting: some studies indicate that vitamin B6 (in yeast, wheatgerm, liver) is vital for hair health, and depletion can lead to falling, thinning hair. Since this nutrient is also depleted by stress, it is no wonder that baldness is often associated with worry. Trichologists say that women are becoming baldies too – so watch out for your B6.
Hair health check list Liver, fish, meat, eggs, yeast, wheatgerm, wholewheat bread, green salads, fresh vegetables, whole grains.

Smooth skin Skin is often the first beauty zone to show signs of ageing horrors! Top requirement for keeping wrinkles at bay (male *and* female ones) is protein – not often a problem, unless you happen to be a vegetarian, in which case you should top up with nuts, lentils and cheese every day. Vitamin C (citrus fruit) is required to help form and maintain collagen – the cement-like material which holds together all the body cells – and gives skin its elasticity and suppleness. You also need vitamins A (carrots, fish liver oils, green vegetables), B complex, especially nicotinic acid, and vitamin D (eggs, milk, butter, sunshine). Vitamin A is depleted if you work under fluorescent lighting, so if your skin is looking spotty, eat more carrots.
Skin health check list Fish, meat, eggs, nuts, lentils, cheese, oranges, lemons, carrots, green vegetables, milk, sunshine.

Bright eyes TV, smoking and booze are death to bright eyes, but diet is even more often to blame for bleariness. Eyes need vitamin A to form 'visual purple', for day and night vision (especially the latter); a deficiency causes eyestrain, soreness, bad vision. Vitamin B2 enzymes normally combine with oxygen to supply the cells in the cornea; where there is a rotten supply, tiny blood vessels form. Get your B2 from yeast, wheatgerm, cheese, liver, kidneys, meat. Eyes also need vitamin C, zinc (sweetbreads, liver, seafoods), and water. Drink plenty if you've consumed a lot of alcohol or feel below par, and try drinking a glass of hot water if you wake up with puffy eyes – this will encourage fluids to drain through the body.
Eye health check list Carrots, leafy greens, yeast, wheatgerm, liver, meat, seafood, water.

Flashing gnashers Teeth need all the above nutrients during growth, plus fluorine to help build up enamel and guard against decay. But once formed, there's precious little you can eat to improve the quality of the teeth you're stuck with. However, you can keep them healthy with crunchy rough-textured foods, and free from decay by avoiding sweet sticky foods. Vitamin C is also very important to help build strong gums ('pink toothbrush' is often a sign of a lack of Vitamin C), as this nutrient is vital for strong capillary walls. Some dentists also believe that bland foods, such as cheese, eaten at the end of a meal can prevent acids from eroding your teeth.

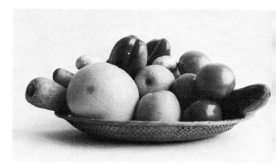

Teeth and gum health check list Raw vegetables, oranges, cheese, water.

Beauty and vitality diet

Here's a seven-day diet to follow when you want to lose some weight and pep up your body. Try it when you feel droopy. It's suitable for anyone in good health (however 'run down' they may be) so if in doubt, consult your doctor. It contains all the good things listed above, and is safe to follow for as long as you need to. You should lose up to 4 lbs in one week.

You may swap around the lunch and supper menus but do not leave out the mid-morning or mid-afternoon snack – this has been carefully planned to curb your appetite for baddies such as sweets, cakes and biscuits. As an extra benefit, buy a bag of wheatgerm and sprinkle it on cereals, salads and fruit salads.

Milk allowance ½ pint a day for use in tea and coffee.
Booze allowance ½ bottle dry wine *or* 2 short drinks with low-calorie mixers *or* 1 pint beer.

Day one
Breakfast 1 orange, 1 cup coffee or tea, 1 crispbread with a little butter and 1 oz Edam cheese.
Mid-morning The juice of 2 lemons and 2 teaspoons of honey mixed in a large glass of hot water.
Lunch 2 egg omelette with 3 grilled tomatoes, coffee or tea.
Mid-afternoon 1 orange.
Supper 4–6 slices of cold chicken without skin, 2 sticks celery, watercress and cucumber with a dressing of 1 teaspoon mustard and juice of half a lemon, coffee or tea.

Day two
Breakfast ½ grapefruit with ½ teaspoon sugar, 1 boiled egg, 1 crisp-bread with a little butter, coffee or tea.
Mid-morning As day one.
Lunch 3 slices corned beef, 2 tablespoons green beans, 2 crisp-breads, 1 oz Edam cheese, coffee or tea.

Mid-afternoon	Other half of morning grapefruit, ½ teaspoon sugar.
Supper	1 bowl low-calorie tomato soup, mixed salad topped with 4 oz grated cheese with dressing of 1 dessertspoon oil and 2 dessertspoons lemon juice, coffee or tea.

Day three

Breakfast	6–8 prunes with 1 chopped apple, 1 tablespoon muesli or similar cereal, coffee or tea.
Mid-morning	As day one.
Lunch	3 lean slices of any cold or hot meat, 2 tablespoons broccoli, 1 apple or pear, coffee or tea.
Mid-afternoon	1 crispbread, butter and 1 oz cheese.
Supper	1 boiled egg, 1 crispbread with butter, large bowl fresh fruit salad, coffee or tea.

Day four

Breakfast	1 bowl stewed apple with honey, 2 lean slices grilled bacon, 1 poached egg, coffee or tea.
Mid-morning	As day one.
Lunch	2 crispbreads and butter topped with 2 oz cheese, tomato, onion and cucumber, coffee or tea.
Mid-afternoon	1 apple.
Supper	2 lean grilled lamb cutlets, grilled mushrooms and tomatoes *ad lib*, 1 tablespoon cauliflower, coffee or tea.

Day five

Breakfast	1 orange, 2 scrambled eggs, 1 crispbread with butter, coffee or tea.
Mid-morning	As day one.
Lunch	3 tablespoons casseroled liver or kidneys, 2 tablespoons any green vegetable, 1 pear, coffee or tea.
Mid-afternoon	1 apple.
Supper	2 crispbreads with butter and 2 oz cheese, 1 natural yogurt, coffee or tea.

Day six

Breakfast	1 bowl fresh fruit salad sprinkled with muesli, coffee or tea.
Mid-morning	As day one.
Lunch	2 grilled sausages with mustard, 1 boiled or baked potato, 1 tablespoon broccoli, 1 fruit yogurt, coffee or tea.
Mid-afternoon	1 bowl fresh fruit salad.
Supper	Grilled fish with lemon, mixed green salad with oil and lemon dressing, 1 crispbread with 1 oz Edam cheese, coffee or tea.

Day seven

Breakfast	1 crispbread with butter and honey, coffee or tea.
Mid-morning	1 natural yogurt.

Lunch	3 slices any roast meat, 1 roast potato, green vegetables, fresh fruit salad, coffee or tea.
Mid-afternoon	Small bunch grapes.
Supper	2 egg omelette, 1 orange with 1 oz Edam cheese, coffee or tea.

The proof of the beauty pudding is in what you really eat! You may have read all my sensible advice on eating for beauty and thought 'yes, but I *know* most of that – so why am I so spotty?' But there's a big difference between knowing what you should eat for your health and good looks and actually *eating* it. A recent survey carried out by the Van den Bergh's food group on what people in Britain eat, revealed that most of us lie in our teeth when asked whether we eat well. When our daily food intake is analysed, meal by meal and snack by snack, the sum total of nutritional value is generally far short of the ideal. It showed for instance that 38 per cent of young unmarried people don't eat breakfast, 15 per cent don't eat lunch and more than half do not eat vegetables with their meals!

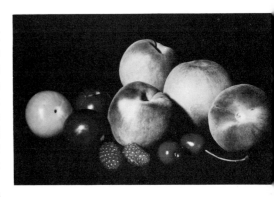

I asked nutritionist Dilys Wells, who helped with the survey, to analyse the daily food intake of a young couple, Kathryn and Michael Daly, aged twenty-one and twenty. The Dalys live in Stevenage, Hertfordshire, and both are office workers; Kathryn is a clerk and Michael is an office manager. Their total food expenditure for the two-week period of surveillance was £64.10, including snacks and drinks.

Here's a typical day's food intake, with comments on each meal from Dilys:

What she ate
Breakfast
4 assorted bisuits

TOTALLY INADEQUATE

Lunch
1 round turkey sandwiches
4 pernod and blackcurrant
NOT ENOUGH PROTEIN

Dinner
shepherd's pie
baked beans
mandarin orange segments

What he ate
Breakfast
2 slices white toast with orange marmalade
1 cup coffee
NOT SUFFICIENT

Lunch
2 sausage rolls
1 pint bitter
POOR NUTRIENT CONTENT

Dinner
shepherd's pie
baked beans
mandarin orange segments

WOULD BE BETTER WITH A FRESH VEGETABLE FOR VITAMIN C; NICER TEXTURE TOO

Between meals:
snacks, drinks, etc.
hamburger and chips
1 twix
1 mars bar
4 coffees
1 cinzano and lemonade
1 pineapple juice
1 snowball

Between meals:
snacks, drinks, etc.
hamburger and chips
4 pints bitter
3 coffees
1 tea

Comments from Dilys Wells The most obvious thing wrong with the Dalys' food is that they eat far too many snacks and drink too much alcohol. Their snacks are of the worst possible sort – chocolate bars, assorted biscuits and similar foods. A likely reason why they eat so many snacks is that their breakfast is inadequate. If they could just eat a little extra protein at breakfast – a boiled egg, slice of cheese or even a glass of milk – they wouldn't want to eat mid-morning.

Many of their lunches too are inadequate. They need to eat more, especially high protein foods like a piece of cheese, or slices of chicken or ham, in addition to their present foods. Their diet would be more nourishing if they were to eat the equivalent calorific value of all those snacks in the form of things like fresh fruit or fruit yogurt or cheese.

Michael drinks a fair amount although it's better he should drink beer than spirits. Kathryn also drinks more than average. The cost of drinks alone could take a large chunk out of the week's food budget. Some of this money could be better spent on more nourishing lunches, fresh fruit, vegetables and salads. I think they should also try brown bread as a change from all white as at present.

Both Kathryn and Michael admit that they sometimes feel tired and droopy. Kathryn suffers from greasy hair occasionally and Michael has dandruff! They are both very beauty and fashion conscious, however, and until the survey was carried out really *didn't* realize how their poor food intake could affect their looks and health. Although neither of them is in poor health they certainly haven't given their bodies a chance to reach their full potential of vitality and attractiveness, both of which are very important qualities for two young people with ambition and a hectic social life. They have decided to take Dilys' advice and modify their diet to include the protein foods, fresh fruit, salads and vegetables which she recommends.

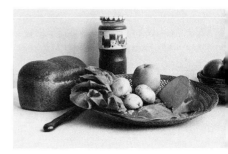

Do have a proper lunch every day – wholemeal bread, a slice of cold meat, raw fruit or vegetables, cheese and fruit juice.

6 Hair Care

Health is the key word when it comes to gorgeous hair. At last, most hairdressers are 'into' hair condition in a big way (if you're reading this after a nightmarish experience at a hairdressing salon not switched on to hair health, then I apologize) and styling is geared to hair type and your life, rather than tortured into the latest fashionable look.

So why do so many of us, male and female, have so many problems with our hair? And why do we spend so much time, money and energy on it? Hairdressing is now such big business that every high street boasts two or three salons and 'crimpers' are the new élite, riding around in limousines and setting up multi-national companies!

The answer to the first question is physical: hair is complex stuff, a body 'barometer' of general health reflecting our hormonal changes and moods; it is also a victim of the amazing things we do to it. It is technically 'dead' material, but it still has this ability to change in various ways and to lead a very active life indeed.

The answer to the second question is psychological: 'mutual grooming' has long been acknowledged by psychologists as a basic human need. We

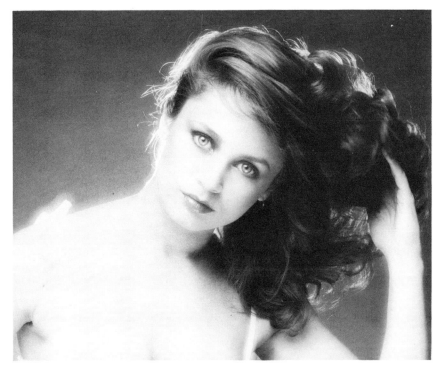

Health is the key word when it comes to a good head of hair.

feel good if we pay someone to cosset, stroke and pamper us; it's as simple as that! Affluence in Western society has transferred the grooming rituals from the home to the salon, and since the huge post-war boom in luxury goods and services, hairdressing establishments are now expanding even further to include beauty departments, manicure, even sauna and massage. It's one aspect of the service industry that doesn't seem to take hard knocks when inflation devalues the cash in your pocket; however hard up you are, you *still* have your hair done! Personally, I feel that good-looking, well-cut hair is a far more valuable beauty asset than a fantastic new outfit or an amazing figure. However busy I am, I always make sure I find time to have my hair cut, permed or coloured when necessary. It boosts my morale more than anything else I know.

What is hair? Hair is made from closely-packed keratin cells . Keratin is a form of protein (the same stuff that makes nails, eyelashes) which is produced by the body from the protein foods we eat. Hair grows at around six inches a year, and everyone (apart from baldies) has around 100,000 hairs on their head.

A section of a single hair, multiplied many thousands of times, is shown in Diagram A. The white outer layer with a scale-like appearance is the transparent cuticle. This is made of flat cells which overlap like roof tiles or fish scales. They act as a protection for the delicate inner layers of the hair. The section in the centre (with the pear-shaped particles) is the medulla, and the layer between the two is called the cortex. The cortex is interesting in that it's here that the colour pigments lie which determine the colour of your hair and it is into this section that permanent colourants or bleaches must penetrate to change the pigmentation chemically. What makes us blondes, brunettes or redheads? We're pre-determined, genetically, to have certain colouring, but the actual substances which do the colouring job in the cortex are formed by a combination of chemicals including melanin and pheomelanin, plus metals. Dark hair is rich in cobalt, copper and iron, red hair is rich in molybdenum, blonde/yellow hair is rich in titanium, and white hair is rich in nickel.

Racial characteristics can also affect hair colour and thickness, as can age. For the technically-minded, the average diameter of an adult human hair is about 70 microns on the Oesterlen scale. Japanese, Chinese and Asians generally have circular hair sections; while Africans have a more flattened hair section and Europeans have an oval-shaped section.

Diagram B shows a close-up of the hair-producing 'factory' in the scalp responsible for the manufacture of each hair. As you can see it's a pretty complex bit of engineering. The grey branch at the base of the diagram is a channel carrying blood to supply life-giving chemicals throughout the body. You can see how it feeds the papilla, the round white object from which the hair is growing. This is the manufacturing plant, deep at the base of the hair. The hair is thicker at the base because it's still soft; as it

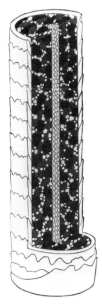

Diagram A.

Diagram B.

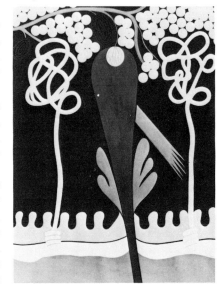

nears the surface it begins to harden and compress, becoming thinner. The frond-like sacs on either side of the hair near the surface of the scalp are the sebaceous glands which supply sebum, an oily substance composed of fatty acids (30 per cent), triglycerides (25 per cent), cholesterol (5 per cent), wax (25 per cent) and hydrocarbons (15 per cent). This substance protects and coats the hair, giving sheen and suppleness. However, if the glands over-supply sebum, then your hair can become too greasy. Similarly, if the sebum is under-supplied it can become dry. Hormonal activity in the body controls the sebum supply, so you can see that hair is very much at the mercy of our general good health and our bodily changes and rhythms.

Damaged hair (Diagram C) looks horrendous under the microscope. Those precious, brilliantly-engineered layers are peeled away and split, the cortex layer weakened or even removed altogether (see small inset diagram). Causes? Harsh chemicals, like strong bleach (especially when successive applications are allowed to overlap), or abusive treatment like over-use of heated rollers and constant brushing. Lack of sufficient protein in the diet will make the hair weak and more susceptible to this kind of damage.

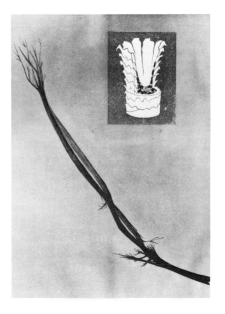

Diagram C.

Diagram D.

Colouring and perming Having a colour change on your hair may be quite a traumatic experience for you, but for your hair it's positively earth-shattering! That's why a good hairdresser will insist that your hair is in pretty good shape before you have a colour change or a perm. There are four main types of colouring products:

Temporary colourants (the kind you buy at the chemist's and use at home or the kind your hairdresser uses to 'brighten up' your hair) deposit colour on the outside of the hair, coating the cuticle. This type of colourant washes out each time the hair is shampooed.

Semi-permanent colourants penetrate just beneath the cuticle and last through about four to six shampoos.

Tints are oxidation dyes made up of chemicals which penetrate into the cortex to deposit colour and they remain in place until the hair grows out. However, sunshine or bodily changes can alter the shade slightly before it grows out.

Double process blonding is a process by which the bleach or lightener strips the pigment from the cortex and another product is used to re-deposit a blonde shade. If you have your hair streaked, then this process is simply applied to small sections of your hair. It does make the hair shaft swell slightly which gives a thicker look and feel to the hair.

Natural colourants such as henna actually coat the hair shaft, but bond on so tightly to the cortex that they, too, must grow out naturally. Henna can be excellent for naturally dark hair which has never been permed or tinted – but is very dodgy indeed for hair which has been treated (see page 109 for the address of a good henna advisory service).

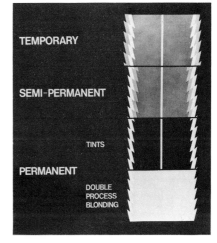

What colour should you choose? Frankly, the colour nearest your own natural colouring is the best bet; it's likely to suit you best (nature is rather good at colour schemes), and will be less of a hassle to keep up. I learned this the hard way by having my naturally dark brown hair tortured into a pale ash blonde for three years with three-weekly visits to the hairdresser to tint out my dark roots. Looking back at old photographs of myself during what I laughingly refer to as my 'Brigitte Bardot' period, I can only say in my defence that I *was* very young. Now I'm a redhead, which suits my freckles and pale skin and involves a three-monthly root and comb-through with a Clairol tint at a London hairdressing salon. I also have a perm every six months and protein treatments in between times if my hair feels dry and looks tacky. If you want to colour your hair at home, use one of the good semi-permanent colourants in a shade near your own and read the instructions carefully before you start. According to the manufacturers about 90 per cent of customers don't bother to read the instructions or do patch or stand tests and then wonder where they've gone wrong. As most of these products do involve a bit of mess, a kind friend is a helpful person to have around while you're coping with the transformation. Bleaching is a dodgy one to try at home unless you have fair hair and can get away with a mild product. In both cases, use a gentle shampoo and lots of conditioner after your colouring treatment to put your hair into a good mood after the traumas.

Perming Perms have made great strides over the last ten years. The chemicals which penetrate the hair shaft, rearranging the molecular structure into a 'curl' shape, are now usually buffered with conditioners and timers which take away some of the hit-and-miss element from the process. A good perm is still largely dependent on a good operator, for it is in the winding and sectioning plus the neutralizing of the hair that the real expertise lies. If the operator gets a series of 'kinks' in your hair, no amount of brushing will remove them. Similarly, if he or she doesn't apply the neutralizer thoroughly (which 'sets' the rearranged hair molecules in place), your perm will droop very quickly.

Two things are necessary when you have a perm: firstly a cut before you have the perm – this is vital to remove as much as possible of the old perm and to get your hair into a good shape for the finished style – and secondly, hair which is in good condition. Never have a perm after a holiday in the sun, when you're feeling tired and under stress, or just before a period. After having a baby, wait until your hair is in good nick again before you perm. Otherwise, you'll be wasting a lot of money!

You can certainly have a perm on tinted hair, but (again!) the hair must be in good condition with no split ends. The perming process will 'lift' the hair colour slightly, so it's best to have your next tint *after* the perm, but not on the same day.

Always allow a full morning or afternoon for your perm and always discuss the style you want fully with the hairdresser before the big day.

Arm yourself with a magazine picture of the kind of thing you want and pop in a week or so before your perm for a consultation. The stylist will tell you whether the style you have in mind is possible for your type/ length/colour of hair and whether it will stand the strain of the experience! Hairdressers complain, quite rightly, that many unsatisfied customers have only themselves to blame for poor results if they insist on breezing into the salon with out-of-condition hair and demand a strong curly perm or a harsh colour change. How do you find a paragon of crimping? One's own Vidal Sassoon is, unfortunately, another's pain in the neck, so recommendation is often the worst way of finding your very own hair-dressing treasure. I have only ever recommended my own hairdresser to two friends: the first said she was grossly overcharged (well, she *did* have streaks, conditioners, and endless cups of coffee), and the second couldn't stand the pop music in the salon! The best thing to do is to go to a salon which boasts about the conditioning treatments they have (Redken or Biothetics franchised salons are all over the country; see end pages for

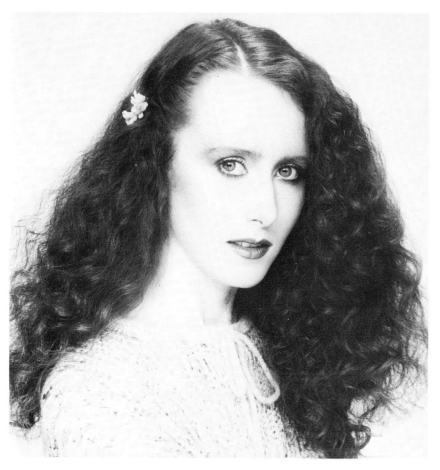

One way to wear long, healthy hair: the hair is plaited when wet, dried thoroughly, then brushed out into masses of tiny pre-Raphaelite waves. Don't pull hair tightly if you plait it when wet – it can stretch up to a quarter of its length.

the head office addresses of both organizations) and explain your requirements. Bear in mind that women are usually quicker, less scissor-happy and more practical about hair styles than men – lovely though male crimpers are! Of course, if your hairdressing requirements are for a confidante and psychologist as well as crimper, then a young trendy male will suit you best (the reverse applies for most men)!

Cutting and styling: can you do your own thing? It is certainly possible to cut your own hair successfully and to do wonders for your family and friends. Trimming fringes, side flicks and the back are all easy to do at home and can save a fortune. However, I suggest that a major change in length and style should be carried out by your hairdresser.

To do a successful haircut at home, you need: scotch tape (the thick opaque kind), very sharp scissors (from a hairdressing supplies wholesaler – see your Yellow Pages), tail comb, straight-backed chair, good mirror (a triple mirror is best if you are cutting your own hair).

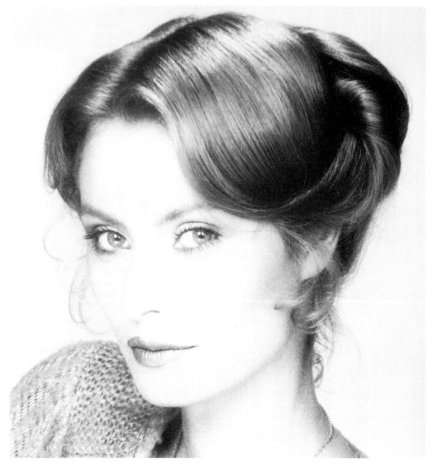

Another way to wear long hair: set it on huge rollers, then part it just off-centre and tuck into a roll at the back, fastened with hair pins. Use tiny heated rollers to curl the wisps round the ears and the nape of the neck.

It is vital to take a long hard look at the hair that is to be cut:
Long hair Is it thick, thin, coarse, fine, straight or curly? If the hair is thick and all one length, check that your scissors are really sharp, otherwise you'll get a very uneven result. Fine, wispy hair also needs the sharp touch. If the hair style is a thick under-turned bob and the texture is coarse, the bottom layer will need to be cut slightly shorter than the top layer to give a bouncy look. Long, naturally curly or permed hair must be cut wet in order to get an even result. Remember that permed hair will look straighter after cutting.
Short hair Check texture carefully and the basic structure of the existing cut. Is it all one length? If not, how many layers is it cut into? Some styles have just three – nape, lower crown and fringe. Others have between four and six layers, or the hair can be cut in short lengths all over the head. Watch out for styles which are cut short at the front, layered on the crown, and left longer at the back.

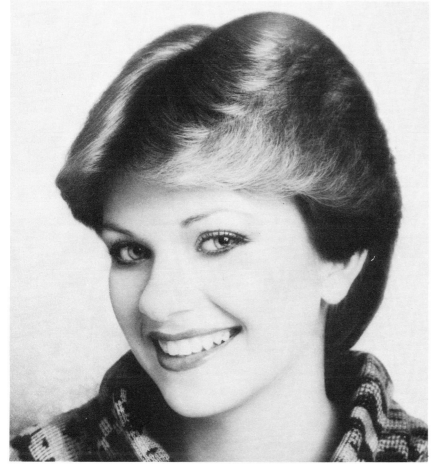

An easy to keep hair style for short hair which can be dried using just your hands under the blow-dryer: the layers are cut short all over but left long enough on top to flick softly away from the face; the edges are shaded slightly darker than the rest to emphasize a strong shape.

Fringes Always tape them in place before you cut, and cut off slightly less than you think you need to! Wet hair is always a bit longer than dry hair.

Moustaches Use a ruler to make each side the same length. If you want to train the moustache into a Viva Zapata droop, cut underneath layers shorter. For a sexy twirl, cut top layers shorter.

Beards Highly personal, like moustaches, these are best trimmed by the owners. While you work check the side view, using two mirrors, as well as the front to make sure the beard looks balanced.

Blunt cut – medium – long hair This cut looks good on straight or wavy hair but the basic hair you are working with must be all one length or long enough to cut to all one length as you work.

1 Wet hair with waterspray. Make a centre parting and comb back hair straight down and front hair forward from the crown. Make a triangular parting across the top of the head with the point in the middle, the two sides running towards the temples.
2 Fasten back hair out of the way with clips, comb fringe section forward. Now place a strip of scotch tape across fringe and cut hair in a straight line just below eyebrow level (it will bounce up when dry). Make sure your line is even.
3 Now cut the back the length you want it along a straight line, first clipping side hair out of the way.

The blunt cut:
Left The fringe is combed forward from a triangular parting (steps 1 and 2).

Centre Cut the back hair before the side hair (steps 3 and 4) and check the length all round.

Below The top layer is clipped up and the underneath layer trimmed a quarter of an inch shorter (step 5) to encourage it to turn under smoothly.

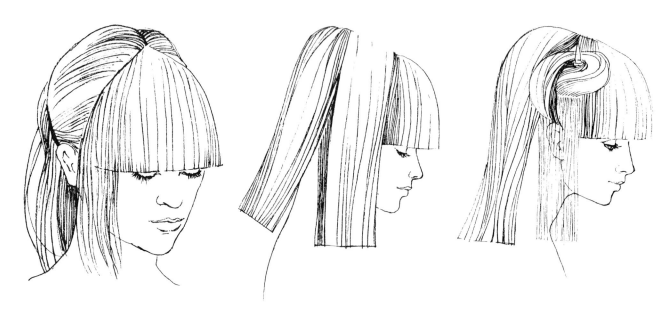

4 Cut left side, then right side in a straight line to match back.

5 Lift up and clip a top layer of side hair away from the main hang of the hair. Cut underneath hair a quarter of an inch shorter, then comb down top hair. Repeat the other side, and at the back.

6 Now check fringe and blow-dry hair using a round styling brush and turning the hair under all the way round (if it is very curly, it will look best allowed to dry naturally).

Tapered cut – short hair This is a good basic cut for short straight hair with a longish front fringe which can be brushed back. The back hair tapers into the nape of the neck.

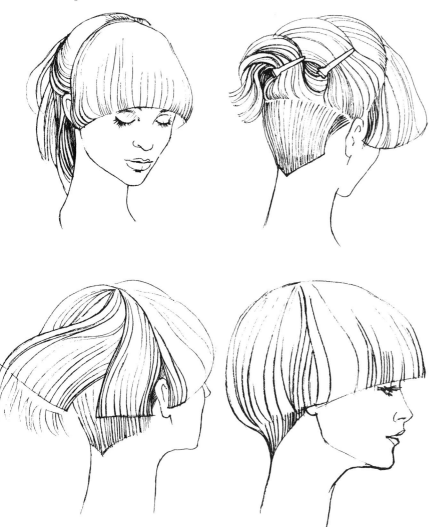

The tapered cut:
Above left The hair is brushed forward and a curved fringe cut from earlobe to earlobe (step 1).

Above right The back hair is clipped up and a deep 'v' cut into the nape of the neck (step 2).

Below left The sectioned-off hair is combed down and cut to earlobe level (steps 3 and 4).

Below right The side hair on a perfect tapered cut should have a 45° slope from the fringe to the nape of the neck (step 5).

1 Brush all hair forward from the crown and dampen thoroughly with waterspray. Now tape hair across forehead and cut a curved fringe from earlobe to eyebrow to the other earlobe. Work in short, even cuts and step back frequently to check your line, constantly combing the hair.

2 Working on the back of the hair, cut a deep 'v' into the nape of the neck, taping the hair first.

3 Remove tape and section off the *top* half of the hair, clipping it out of the way. Replace tape on nape 'v' and re-check the line.

4 Now work on the sectioned-off hair, cutting it to earlobe level straight across the back.

5 Remove tape, comb down sides of the hair and lift a small section each side of the earlobe. Trim an extra quarter of an inch off the underneath hair after taping. Remove tape, comb down hair and check that line – it should make a 45° slope from the forehead down to the nape of the neck. Check the other side.

6 Make a centre parting, and blow-dry hair, flicking back the sides of the fringe.

Blow-drying This can be very harmful if you use a strong blast of hot air against your hair (lots of hairdressers get their juniors to do blow-drying – if your hair is overheated in this callous way, *complain*). Hold your dryer six inches away from your hair and brush hair from the root at an angle of 90° to the scalp for maximum bounce. Always start with crown hair and work down to fringe and back hair. There is no need to blow-dry hair from soaking wet; always dry off the excess moisture first to prevent arm-ache. Don't tug or you'll over-stretch your hair (it can stretch to about 25 per cent of its own length when wet – but then snap!). Your brush should be firm but soft, not scratchy. There are several good shampoos on the market specially for blow-dried hair. If you repeat this tough performance several times a week you *must* use a mild shampoo and condition your hair regularly. Personally, I'm rather 'anti' too much blow-drying. Rollers are kinder to the hair.

Roller-setting Again, dry off excess moisture first and set your hair carefully, holding each section at a 90° angle to the scalp. The best rollers are the lightweight plastic ones – don't use metal rollers (they overheat the hair shaft), or bristle ones (they tangle and break the hair). If you can, let roller-set hair dry naturally or sit under a hooded dryer. Don't be tempted to speed up the drying process by holding your dryer too near your hair.

Quickie styling tips
Rolling and plaiting For a fashionable look with long hair, make a centre parting and roll up back hair, fastening with hair pins. Set front wisps in tiny pin-curls. This looks very pretty and romantic, and works well if your

hair is a bit 'tacky' and you don't have time for a shampoo. Tiny plaits on the crown or sides of the hair can be caught up with slides or flowers for a charming 'milkmaid' effect, or a front section simply twisted back and fastened with a flower or clip. If you wish, all-over plaiting can be done when hair is wet (after a shower or swim perhaps). Later the plaits brush out to a delicious pre-Raphaelite mass of hair (picture on page 35).

Gel styling On short hair, you can try a fabulous and dramatic look using (wait for it!) gynaecological jelly. This gel is water-soluble so washes out very easily, unlike greasy hairdressings. Simply smother hair in gel and shape into pin-curls and deep 'twenties waves with old fashioned wave clips. This look is marvellous on short dark hair with dramatic eye make-up and clothes. On holiday, use a protective product in much the same way. Several manufacturers now have 'barrier' dressings which help to protect the hair from the sun and sea. Smother hair with barrier cream (such as Parasol by Molton Brown) in the morning, push into waves or slick back under a scarf or hat and wash out again in the evening.

Scarves Long scarves look good plaited together and bound round the head, leaving the back hair hanging loose or hiding the hair altogether if it's in need of a wash or trim.

The French pleat This 'fifties favourite is back in fashion again and is easy to style: simply brush hair to one side, make a row of grips up the centre back of the hair, brush hair back, roll under and fasten with hair pins. The front hair can be curled or swept back, or just fastened back with a stylish slide or flower.

Going thin on top? Falling hair hits most of us at some time or other – after all, the least we can expect to lose is about eighteen to twenty hairs a day, even when we're in perfect health. The crunch for many women comes after the birth of their first child: the glossy mane which shone serenely through nine months of pregnancy suddenly becomes a lank, thin, pathetic mess. Blame hormonal activity, nutritional depletion (your vitamins and minerals are now bouncing around in the baby!) and natural stress and anxiety. A senior trichologist at London's Scalp and Hair Hospital (address on page 112) says: 'With each pregnancy, a woman's hair gets a little thinner, even though there is a certain amount of recovery after each baby. Pregnancies which are close together are particularly bad for the hair – it just doesn't have a chance to get growing again.'

Dyes, perms, bleaching and straightening (the worst offender of the lot) cause a certain amount of breakage and falling hair. A bad hairdresser or a do-it-yourself job which involves dye or bleach overlap on the hair shaft will make the hair root brittle and likely to snap. It's almost impossible to wait for a perm to grow out completely before having the next one, but it is wise to have as much 'end' cut off as possible to avoid the dreaded fall-out. Straightening is a baddie because the lotion is often just as harsh as a perming chemical and is usually placed directly against the root of the

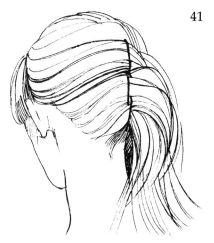

To make a neat French pleat, brush hair firmly to one side and fix it with a vertical line of hairgrips worked up from the nape to the crown.

Brush hair over the hairgrip line and roll under. Fasten it with hair-matched pins, *not* grips (they will make the roll look flat and clumsy). Any straggly ends can be smoothed down with a light hairspray.

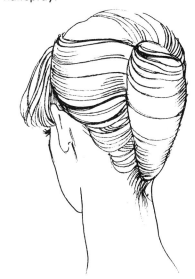

hair and consequently against the scalp too. As the kinks and curls start growing again, more straightening lotion is applied, and some of it is bound to run down the hair shaft to weaken the already straightened hair.

Permanent hair-dyeing using oxidation dyes (the kind used for tinting at most hairdressers – see page 109) doesn't necessarily weaken the hair, but if the re-touching is badly done or you swap colours frequently, it can cause unnecessary hair loss. The best idea is to go for a colour near your own so the minimum amount of chemical action is needed. Fine hair should never be subjected to monthly bleaching and tinting – if you want to keep it.

Blow-drying is another horror. If the dryer is held close to the hair shaft, the tiny overlapping keratin particles will be forced apart, dried out and eventually snap. If the hair is brushed repeatedly (never a good thing for hair – sorry, granny, your hundred strokes were a rotten idea) and dragged unmercifully into shape it will look great for the short time before you have to invest in a wig!

The patchy kind of alopecia where just a few hairs, or a small patch of hair, fall out is caused in about 90 per cent of cases by stress or shock, and this is an increasing problem among women. The shock might be anything from running over the neighbour's cat to having an almighty row with the boss. The body reacts in a very sneaky way to shock: antibodies which usually protect us from germs and other nasties, turn on us instead; they cause symptoms like eczema, dermatitis, shingles and clumps of falling hair. The shock can be a delayed reaction to a series of events too: for example, taking a demanding job, then losing a close relative, and finally splitting up with your husband. It's easy to say 'avoid stress and you'll keep your hair on', but darned hard to put into practice. Taking holidays – short, frequent ones are best – devoting time to a sport or hobby, learning to keep your cool under pressure; these can all help. There is also no substitute for security, both financial and emotional. Those society beauties with glossy manes of hair never have to worry about where the next shampoo and set is coming from, which must contribute to their abundant coiffures. Love is cheaper and equally good for the hair.

In most cases hair which falls out after one of these traumas does grow again. Scalp care is essential to encourage the new growth. Hair follicles which are blocked by dandruff or oily deposits can impede the progress of the new hairs. A qualified trichologist is the best person to treat the condition; he will usually prescribe special shampoos, massage lotions, Vitamin B tablets and iron. But do consult an expert if you have this trouble, through your doctor if you like, or see the addresses on page 112.

Total baldness is still comparatively rare among women. It's programmed to occur in men way back during puberty when a hormone called testosterone comes swinging into action producing sex drive, genital hair growth, beard growth, etc. While it's doing all that, it occasionally has one negative effect: it causes hair to start thinning out. Women have very little testosterone activity during puberty, but later, during the menopause, they often tend to go thin on top because of lack of another hormone, oestrogen. The combination of the menopause and crises, with teenage offspring or husband going off the rails, is highly conducive to baldness.

One growing problem in younger women is falling hair which is not adequately replaced in the natural way simply because anaemia is present. This can be due to improper diet (the buns, cakes and chips routine) so it is worth examining your eating habits carefully if you are a young thin-on-top lady. Healthy blood feeds the new hairs in the follicle and you can find iron in meat (liver, kidneys – eat one or the other twice a week), eggs, leafy greens like watercress, spinach and cabbage. Hair is made from protein, so an adequate supply of that is obviously necessary. If you're living mainly on starch, step up meat, cheese, fish and milk, and cut out the padding.

Covering the evidence of a bad baldness attack is simpler for women than it is for men. Female-type wigs look less 'wiggy' than the male type. I have yet to see a male wig which doesn't look obvious because of the join line at the front of the scalp. However, wigs are becoming very fashionable indeed for men these days – the TV newscasters seem to go for them in a big way! If your bald patch is very tiny or you have thinning hair on top, a light perm can make the hair look thicker and help cover the spot (men are going overboard for perms too, especially footballers!).

Hair transplants can be successful, although costly and time-consuming. You have to be prepared to wear a hat for some time to cover the scars on top while the hair is 'taking'. If you're in show business or are sufficiently extrovert not to mind the comments, then the time and money may be a good investment. However, a qualified trichologist will tell you if you're likely to be the right material for a transplant. It's wise to check first before you get involved with a transplant surgeon – the trichologist may be able to recommend a good surgeon for you.

7 Smile Please

Or, on second thoughts, don't. For if you do bare your molars in a seductive grin, the chances are that they will let your image down with a horrible bang. The vast majority of people in this country have appalling teeth. A recent survey by the British Dental Association revealed that 30 per cent of adults have lost all their teeth, more than half have some false teeth and 95 per cent of us have signs of gum disease.

Yet it's comparatively easy to keep our teeth and gums healthy and prevent disease and decay. So why don't we bother? It isn't just that we're a nation of sweet-eaters (although that doesn't exactly help the problem), it's also the fact that we just don't clean our teeth properly. In the same survey, the British Dental Association found that one toothbrush in three is virtually useless. Apathy, and the idea that dentists are paid to take care of our teeth for us, is the root cause of the bad state of the nation's molars. From the beauty and health point of view, it's worth remembering that tooth and gum troubles don't just cause localized problems, they can also

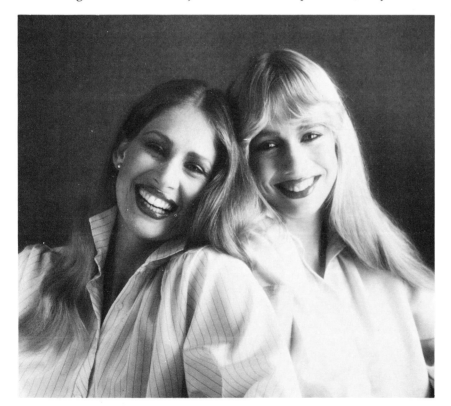

There is no excuse for bad teeth nowadays, so *do* look after them — and keep smiling!

trigger off stomach complaints, digestive problems, earache, headaches and sickness. Here's what you should know about your teeth – and what you should be doing to look after them:

Teeth and gum care Dentists say that more teeth are lost through gum disease than through decay itself. Unhealthy gums just can't support your teeth, so they literally fall out.

What causes disease? Plaque, the invisible bacterial film continuously forming on the teeth actually soaks into the gums if it isn't completely removed every twenty-four hours. The plaque build-up eventually hardens, starts to calcify and becomes calculus (tartar) which causes inflammation and eventually deepens the crevice between the tooth and gum. Then, the bone supporting the tooth and gum structure starts to wear away and the tooth becomes loose. You can tell if your teeth are in danger by looking at your gums: healthy gums are pale pink, firm and have a texture like orange peel; inflamed gums are red, often shiny and bleed easily, especially when you clean your teeth. If yours are like this, then you should throw out your old toothbrush, and choose one with a medium-sized head and multi-tufted with round-ended nylon filaments. It should be soft or medium – hard toothbrushes cause abrasion and damage. Brush teeth and gums in short, deliberate strokes concentrating on the area where the gum meets each tooth. Brush the same surface many times using a three-minute egg-timer to make sure you give your teeth the attention they deserve. Backs *and* fronts! Use softwood sticks or dental floss to clean the narrow gaps between the teeth; both are available at chemists. The floss should be wound between the second fingers of each hand, grasped by the finger and thumb and then gently passed between the teeth; push down the side of each tooth in a gentle up-and-down movement. Use between all teeth, not just the front ones.

What about toothpaste? Most dentists recommend toothpaste containing fluoride to help strengthen teeth, but remember that the brushing itself is your most important cleaning device. Don't put too much paste on the brush, otherwise you'll spend more time foaming at the mouth and spitting in the sink, than actually brushing your teeth.

After a week of this treatment, you'll notice that your gums and teeth will look healthier and feel less tingly and sore. If necessary, back up the treatment with a visit to your dentist for the removal of calculi and a practical demonstration of just how to brush your teeth. Pregnancy weakens the resistance of the gums to disease, so extra care is needed to keep them plaque-free. Gum resistance can also weaken in women taking the Pill. It's also a side-effect if you're on a daft, unbalanced slimming diet, or are 'run down', or otherwise low and droopy.

Tooth decay prevention Dental decay occurs when the enamel protecting the teeth is eaten away until a hole is made. Causes? Plaque again, often

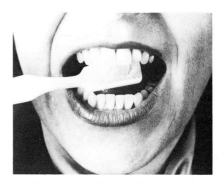

Don't forget the back of your teeth when you clean them. Your toothbrush should be like the one shown here: medium head, rounded end, fine nylon filaments – and not more than three months old.

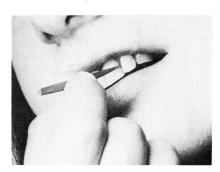

A softwood stick can help clean between your teeth. Moisten the pointed end, insert between the teeth with the flat edge next to the gum, then use a gentle in-out motion to clean between the teeth. Don't prod. You can also use dental floss to do the same job.

when there is the additional 'load' of sugar. Plaque thrives on sugar and actually uses it to produce the strong acid that destroys tooth enamel. It's vital to control your sugar intake and avoid all sticky foods that cling to the teeth: toffees, biscuits, sweet puddings and confectionery. It's better to eat sugary foods (if you must) all at once, after a meal perhaps, than continuously throughout the day. *Always* brush your teeth thoroughly after a meal. Acid can also erode tooth enamel; taking neat lemon juice every day isn't a good idea for this reason. Try to end a meal with a bland food such as cheese rather than an apple. As far as fluoride preparations are concerned, this is a matter for personal choice. However, dentists are certainly in favour of them, from tablets to toothpastes. It is certainly true, though, that they are more effective for children than adults.

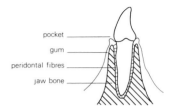

The root of the tooth is suspended in the bone by the peridontal fibres which are attached to the root surface and the bone itself.

Cosmetic dentistry If, after all your care, it's necessary to lose a tooth, what can be done other than resorting to a 'falsie' or a gap? More and more people are now spending time and money on cosmetic dentistry to correct congenital dental faults and patch-up problems – including the loss of teeth. According to the amount of damage, a tooth can be 'crowned' (filed down to a stump, when a metal peg is inserted into the root and a 'crown' of porcelain fixed on top) or replaced altogether by a 'bridge' of one or more porcelain teeth which is anchored to sound teeth either side of the gap. The porcelain teeth are carefully colour-matched to the natural teeth, and look extremely realistic. However, these treatments are only available on the National Health Service where there is real need, although some dentists who enjoy this kind of work seem to be able to get cosmetic problems 'passed' by the Dental Estimates Board, who control the pounds and pence, much more easily than others.

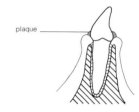

Plaque is a colourless film of bacteria which builds up round the top of the gum and causes inflammation.

If you have to pay out for cosmetic dentistry, the cost can certainly be high; anything from £50 for a single crown to £2,000 plus for a mouthful of problems. However, it certainly may be a good investment in terms of your looks and general health. First, get an estimate of cost, time (and pain, if you're a coward) from a reputable dentist. How to find one? This can be a problem although your National Health dentist should be able to recommend someone if he or she doesn't do private cosmetic work. It is certainly worth going to someone who is a specialist in this kind of work and who has the back-up of the technicians who produce the crowns and plates and do the 'artwork' necessary for a convincing result.

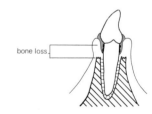

The plaque has calcified and formed a pocket between the tooth and gum.

Dentures If you wear dentures, do check that they fit correctly, as the structure of the mouth and gums can alter with time causing discomfort. Clean with a soft brush and soap or toothbrush, after all meals if possible. Dentists prefer you to remove them at night as the underlying mouth tissue can rest and come into contact with the flow of saliva, but if you can't face sleeping with a 'gummy' look, try to 'rest' your mouth at some other time during the day – while you bath, perhaps.

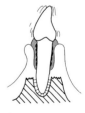

The bone has been completely worn away and the tooth is ready to fall out.

8 Bosom Pals

Why are we all so hung up about our breasts? Most beauty writers (including me) get more letters about bosom beauty than any other part of the female anatomy. According to psychologists, the feminine preoccupation with breasts is part vanity, part natural protectiveness. 'They're the most important symbol of a woman's femininity,' says one, 'and her most valuable asset for successfully rearing her offspring. Her breasts are sexy, sensual, sensitive, registering hormonal changes inside her body – no wonder she thinks about them so often!'

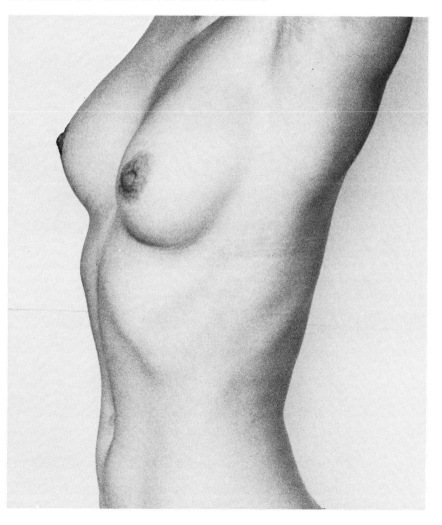

A good bosom depends as much on deportment as on diet and exercise.

We're now bombarded with so many pictures of Miss Superboob in magazines and newspapers that our own humble offerings seem even less desirable than in the good old days when anyone could fake a good cleavage with brown eye shadow and sticky tape. Now, clothes are so skimpy and revealing that you simply can't wear a bra with most of them, particularly the summer kind. Droops, sags and odd bulges show, so do huge floppy bosoms and funny little boyish ones. No wonder so many women are 'into' the whole idea of plastic surgery for the bosom beautiful . . . and no wonder so many surgeons are making so much money out of it!

I believe that there's a lot you can do to improve the look of your bosom, even though changing the size involves something radical like a pregnancy or mammoplasty (this reduces giant bosoms)! Here are some bosom care facts:

Your bosom – structure and care Each breast is a squashy mound of fat tissue used as a protective covering to milk producing glands. It's given 'uplift' by a pair of pectoral muscles, situated slightly above and to one side of each breast. These muscles have a lot of work to do, since there is nothing supporting the bosom underneath. Therefore, the larger your breasts, the stronger your pectorals need to be to support you in an 'uplifting' position. Wearing a bra if you're bigger than a size 34 B isn't old-fashioned – it's vital. However if you wear skimpy clothes, you should try to give your bosom some support by changing into a sensible shirt or T-shirt every other day, and wearing a light bra. Young breasts will sag alarmingly if not supported during pregnancy, so do wear a bra then. It also helps relieve the load on your pectorals if you sit and stand with shoulders well back, but relaxed. Hunched shoulders will make the dreaded droops even worse.

Try these two exercises for strengthening the pectoral muscles:

1 Stand or sit, arms by your sides. Now slowly raise your arms sideways to a point halfway between shoulders and head. Now slowly draw your arms forward, feeling your pectorals work hard as you do so. Stop just before your arms touch, and pull your shoulder blades together towards your spine, forcing your arms apart. Lower arms, relax muscles. Repeat slowly five times.
2 Sitting comfortably (at work perhaps), bring your arms up in front of you, bend your elbows and grab your left forearm with your right hand, your right forearm with your left. Without moving your hands push sharply (feel your breasts rising?), hold for a count of six, then relax. Repeat as often as possible.

These exercises are particularly necessary when you're on a slimming diet. You may lose weight in the breast area very quickly and you'll sag there if you're not careful.

49

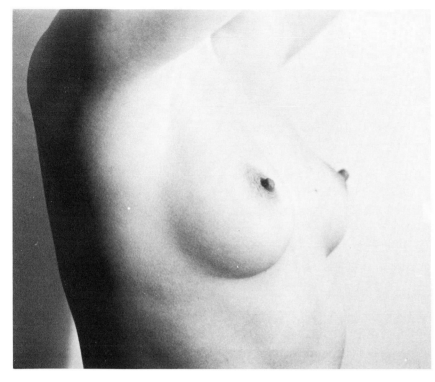

A tiny bosom can look firm and
shapely if you practice
breast-firming exercises regularly.
Small bosoms are equally efficient
for breast-feeding too!

What about creams and lotions? Several firms now produce perfectly
harmless creams and lotions for bosom conditioning and firming. These
are based on natural plants and herbs and don't contain hormones.
However, I think their value is limited to firming the actual skin . . . not
the basic structure. Gravity and muscular control are the important factors there. But these creams do have a soothing and softening effect on
delicate tissue and are very useful during pregnancy when bosom beauty
and care is very important.

Bosoms and motherhood Nourish the skin of your rapidly growing bust-
line with creams and lotions (see above) and rub nipples with baby oil,
'twiddling' with thumb and forefinger if you want to breast-feed. Supple
nipples are more important than the size of your equipment. Towards the
end of your pregnancy, you *must* wear a specially-made supporting bra if
your bosom reaches mammoth proportions. But watch your diet during
pregnancy; you don't need more calories, just more nutrients! Zinc (in
seafood and green vegetables) is important to prevent stretch marks.

　　After the baby is born, breasts really come into their own (after all, this
is what they've been waiting for!), and go hard and rigid as the colostrum
and the milk start to rush in. Feeding is good for your tummy muscles, but
can be a strain on your breasts and can leave you with less than you had

before. Sit upright when you feed, don't lean forward, and wear a good bra (cotton) at all times. Those flimsy numbers will just have to wait for a few months. After feeding is over, do the exercises above regularly. If you have stretch marks (and you shouldn't if you've taken the advice above), then a Vitamin E cream can help fade them.

Breast cosmetic surgery If, after all the care above, you hate your bosom and it's making your life a misery, then breast augmentation or mammoplasty are certainly readily available. Expect to pay about £400 for an augmentation operation, £700 for mammoplasty. Here's what they entail:

Augmentation An incision is made under the breast and a small bag containing soft silicone jelly is placed between the chest wall and the under-surface of the breast gland making the breast move upwards and outwards. The incision is then stitched up. Obviously, the size of the silicone bag depends on how many extra inches you want and this in turn is governable to a great extent by the amount of tissue and skin available. The operation involves a three-day stay in a clinic.

Mammoplasty This is a more complicated operation where the breasts are actually re-moulded, tissue is removed and the skin tightened. The nipple may be moved to a higher position to make it firmer and perkier. The amount of scarring depends on the size of the problem but there is usually more scarring than with the augmentation operation where the small scar fits neatly under the fold of the breast. The operation involves five days or so in the clinic with a six-week post-operative recovery period. Some surgeons insist that patients should be under fifty for this op.

Post-mastectomy reconstruction More surgeons are now performing remarkable reconstruction jobs on breasts removed by mastectomy operations. However, the success of these is determined by the extent of the mastectomy operation and the patient's own willingness to be 'messed about' after such radical surgery. Nipples and skin can be re-formed from the patient's own body – grafting from the buttocks and just outside the lips of the vagina for the nipples. It is now possible for some patients to have this done on the National Health Service, although surgeons sometimes advise a wait between mastectomy and reconstruction. However, they do say that there's more chance of a successful implant operation if the malignant growth is caught early ... which is yet one more reason for regular manual breast checks and yearly screening examinations.

9 Hands, Knees and Boomps-a-daisy

Three very vulnerable, sensitive and deserving body areas are often forgotten in the wear and tear of everyday life, but all three respond brilliantly to pampering. The areas? Hands and nails, knees – and bottoms! Hands are neglected by the fussiest people; nails bitten down to the quick, skin rough and red, cuticles tattered and torn. Knees are hard, scaly and even grimy. Bottoms are spotty (men are the main sufferers here), saggy, or red and flabby! Here's how to revitalize all three trouble spots.

Hands and nails Paint stripper, chemical cleaners, axle grease, detergents, typing, coping with kids, stress, nervous tension – the list of things which ruin your hands is endless. You can't expect 'miracle' nail-lengthening creams to help, if the basic raw material is devoid of nourishment. For, like all aspects of beauty care, nail and hand beauty starts from *within*. Nails are made from closely-packed keratin cells; they also contain smaller amounts of calcium, phosphorus and trace metals. Nails need protein, Vitamin A and iron for healthy growth. Protein sources are meat, fish, eggs and cheese, and if you cut down on these (on a slimming diet for instance), your nails will break, split and peel. Vitamin A is less easy to obtain in your diet than protein, as it is supplied by liver, fish liver oils, egg yolk, butter and cream, and manufactured in the body from the yellow pigment, carotene, found in carrots, apricots and parsnips. If your nails peel easily or become ridged, the chances are that you're not getting your fair share of this vitamin. If you have little white spots in your nails, then you could be zinc-deficient; good sources are cheese, eggs, liver, oysters and herring. This mineral is vital during pregnancy – herring are a good source of vitamin D too, so step up your intake of delicious grilled herring. Mild anaemia (iron deficiency) produces brittle fingernails with longitudinal ridging and most women suffer from iron deficiency during menstruation.

Hands do have natural protection in the form of oils and sweat, but, naturally, we wash that off as often as possible! If you want to keep soft hands don't worry about the brand of detergent you use or your washing up liquid, just never *ever* let your hands come into contact with either of them! Rubber gloves may not be glamorous but they are essential wearing for every woman or man with dirty jobs to tackle. Men may scoff at the very idea of wearing gloves to wash the car, but soft hands are certainly sexier to the touch than calloused, hard ones. Barrier creams can help if the job is so sensitive that gloves simply cannot be worn. You can make up a good one by mixing one teaspoon kaolin with one teaspoon almond oil and the yolk of one egg. Work the mixture into hands and under nails. Allow to dry thoroughly. Wash off when your work is finished. Always use handcream after bathing or washing and keep a tube handy in the kitchen, car and office desk. I also keep a tube by my bedside and apply it just before I go to sleep which gives an eight-hour beauty treatment to my hands.

Do you do a potentially nail-breaking job? Then keep your nails fairly short and file them in an oval shape. Typing with long nails is uncomfortable and hazardous; bricklaying is the same. Don't imagine that commercial nail conditioners will prevent nail breakage if you don't wear a protective polish on top. These products simply soften the nail and surrounding skin; they may contain a very small amount of protein which will give a more flexible and glossier look to the topmost keratin layers of the nail but protein is really more use inside your body. Protect your nails with nail polish (most contain nylon or a similar strengthening ingredient now) and use two or three coats topped by a vinyl-based protective coat if you like – they are only marginally tougher than an extra coat of the polish itself and no miracle worker if you intend to decoke your Range Rover. It's a good idea, whatever the product, to paint the nail over the tip and underneath it too.

Check your nail polish every night and top with an extra coat until you have to re-do the lot. It's most practical to wear a colour that 'goes' with everything you wear as changing nail varnish daily is a chore for the idle rich only! Scarlet, plum and rust are good basics.

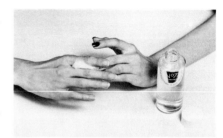
Removing old polish.

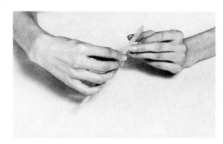
Filing nails, sides towards centre.

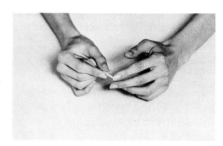
Cleaning nails.

The Do-it-Yourself Manicure

Here's a foolproof manicure guide for busy people. Men can use clear varnish if they wish.

1 Remove old polish with a gentle nail polish remover. Look for one with lanolin or other softening formula. Hold cotton wool between the first two fingers of one hand and rub one nail at a time against it.
2 Dabble fingertips in soapy water (bland soap, not detergent!), dry and then file into an almond shape. Use an emery board, and file in one direction from sides towards centre. Never file too low at the sides.
3 Clean underneath nails with the pointed end of an orange stick. If they are filthy, wrap a bit of cotton wool soaked in cuticle remover around the stick before tackling the dirt.
4 Apply cuticle remover lotion or cream along the base and sides of your nails. Leave for five minutes, then gently push the cuticle back with the blunt end of the stick. Wash hands, then massage in a nail conditioning

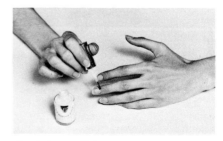
Applying cuticle remover.

52

cream or hand cream, rubbing well into the matrix or growth area of the nail below the half-moon. The action will stimulate blood flow to the area, and help with growth.

5 Prepare nail surface for polish by dabbling nails into a weak solution of lemon juice (one teaspoonful juice to one cup water).

6 Apply strengthener if you use it. Cover the back of the nail as well as the front.

7 Now apply one or two coats of polish, plus a top coat if you like. The strokes should be from root to tip, centre first, then either side. Try to leave a good ten minutes between coats. TV programmes are really good for 'timing' your nail varnish: allow one commercial break for each coat!

Falsies and filling treatments If you are a nail biter then false nails can help you kick the habit and give your own nails a fighting chance of growing. Alternatively, use an anti-bite product which tastes nasty, and arm yourself with delicious, scrunchy apples which will do you good while they help you beat the nail-nibbling problem. Quite a few nail-rebuilding studios have opened up around the country where artificial, semi-permanent nails can be fixed to your own. However, this process can occasionally damage the nail which has to be buffed to take the fixative used. The finished nails last for two weeks and certainly do look good.

Knees that please Do you have knees that look like over-cooked rock-cakes, or are yours more like squashy doughnuts? Either way it's a shame! The skin on knees (and elbows and ankles) contains fewer sebaceous glands than other parts of the body so they do dry out very easily. Spare a moment to massage and pummel them at bathtime, lavishing lots of creams and lotions on their poor dry, parched skin. Avoid kneeling directly on the floor to do a chore; use a cushion instead. If knees become grimy, then wash gently with a soft nail brush using circular movements and bland soap before your bath. One manufacturer makes a special hard skin treatment cream which is applied before the bath and leaves knees feeling silky-smooth and looking good. Puffy knees? This problem is known among beauticians as the 'air hostess syndrome', since air stewardesses seem to suffer from it. It also afflicts all regular jet travellers. Why? Biologically, the answer lies in *fluid retention*, the common beauty problem consistently dismissed by doctors as female nonsense. For some reason, pressurized cabins seem to cause pockets of fluid to lodge around the knees instead of their other little favourite spots: tummy, hips and thighs. Diuretic foods such as oranges and lemons can help encourage the fluids to leave the body in a decent fashion via urine. Drink extra water but cut out fluid-trapping coffee, tea and milky drinks. Carbohydrate foods will soak up fluid like a sponge too. Cut out cakes, biscuits and spuds and concentrate on protein and leafy greens. Sit with your feet up, literally: bottom against a wall, legs stretched up it. Do this every night after work.

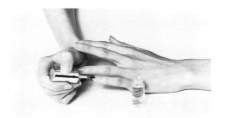

Nail strengthener helps protect the nail tip.

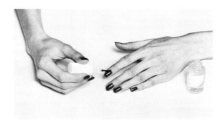

A high gloss coat gives extra shine.

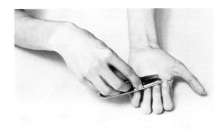

Use a chamois buffer if you don't wear polish.

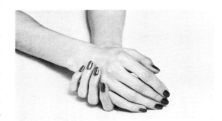

The finished manicure.

Make-up for knees? Why not. Leg make-up can be a good idea if yours are grey-looking or white in summer. Try rosy blusher on your knees to make them glow. Apparently, as with earlobes, glowing knees can be a subtle sexual signal. The mind boggles!

Bottoms Do you know what your bottom looks like or are you afraid to ask your best friend? Most of us are all too aware of our bulges and sags in other areas but afraid to face up to the awful truth about our backsides (if you know what I mean). Buttocks, those soft twin pads of flesh, are potentially very beautiful indeed but are often allowed to fall into disrepair. Here's how to make the most of your bot:

Toning up the muscles Bottoms are soft and squashy, and they need muscle tone to become taut and rounded. If you sit on a cushion or soft chair while you work, watch TV or drive, your muscles will quickly become slack, and flab will be encouraged to build up around them. So, throw away the cushions, sit up straight and practise contracting your buttock muscles hard for a count of six whenever you have to sit still for long periods. I'm convinced that this simple excercise has prevented my own thirty-six-inch posterior from spreading, despite the years of being chained to my typewriter in a sitting-down position! I do this exercise frequently throughout the day, even when I'm waiting for a bus or sitting in the train. It doesn't show, honestly! I have also encouraged others in sitting-down jobs to try it, including a few MPs! Walking, with healthy, long strides, is also good bottom muscle exercise. So is this one: lie face down on the bed or floor, lift your left leg as high as you can, cross it over your right leg and lower. Raise again; lower back to starting point. Repeat with the other leg.

Avoid constricting your bottom in too-tight jeans or skirts; they will prevent your muscles from actually working at the job they are meant to do. They can also produce a dangerous squashing of fatty tissue at thigh level resulting in 'cellulite' fatty deposits which are very hard to get rid of. If you have funny bumps and bulges together with a grey-looking sluggish skin colour and 'orange peel' texture, then you must combine a programme of massage with a good diet.

Try pinching, twisting and pummelling the flesh on your thighs and buttocks with your fingers under warm bathwater. This will take the agony out of the process while helping to encourage circulation (those jeans have probably made your poor bot forget all about its blood supply). Your diet should be similar to the puffy knees one above: oranges, lemon tea, lots of water (preferably mineral water, the still kind not the fizzy kind) and protein foods. Cut out stodge, booze and fried foods for a while at least. You'll find that the improvement will be slow but sure. You can also try rubbing an infusion of ivy leaves into the offending area. This isn't as quaint as it sounds since ivy extract is renowned for its localized diuretic and softening properties (indeed one French beauty house

Bottoms are tops! A small, neat bottom looks good dressed and undressed.

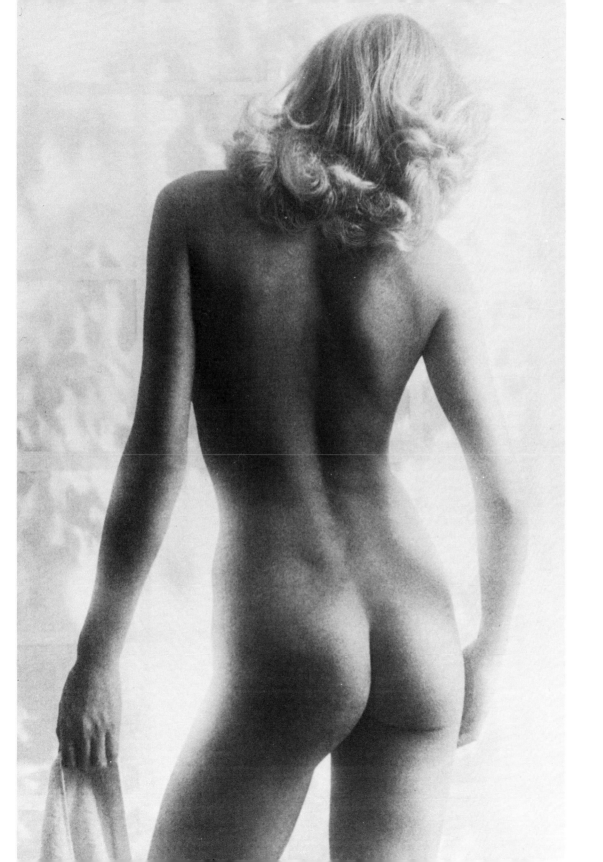

produces a special ivy-based lotion especially for puffy bots and thighs).
Pick a bundle of ivy leaves to fill a two-pint saucepan loosely, tear them up roughly and simmer in two pints of boiling water for fifteen minutes. Strain the liquid and rub it into your bottom and thighs every night before your bath, using a loofah or bath mitt.

Getting rid of spots Spotty bot is a driver's hazard especially if he or she drives on plastic car-seats wearing nylon pants. Clean the area carefully every night, use a spot-drying preparation and wear cotton undies. Sunbathe nude or use a lamp to help dry the skin. In fact, nudity is a good treatment for this problem and practical if you live in a secluded area.

Dealing with roughness If your bottom is dry and rough try adding a capful of baby oil to your bathwater plus a tablespoonful of cider vinegar. Massage with body lotions or even a nourishing face cream. If rough skin is a general problem look to your diet. Step up liver, take yeast tablets and add vegetable oils to your salads to help boost your sebaceous glands' supply of protective body oil. Stress is also one cause of dry skin and eczema, so try to relax more too.

10 Underneath the Arches

They may be a long way away, but feet have feelings! This is a fact which is often painfully underlined when nasty twinges contort your face with agony while you're running (running? – more like hobbling) for a bus. Exceptionally tall people and pregnant mums have been known to forget about feet altogether for some months, but even they are rapidly brought down to earth when the screaming abdabs start. Beauty pundits like me are always saying 'if your feet hurt, it shows on your *face*' which is a boring thing to say because it's so true! Ill-fitting shoes, pointed toes and lack of instep support are the three top causes of foot deformities. Bad or non-existent nail trimming, poor hygiene and sweaty socks or tights are the three top causes of horrors like soft corns, soreness and in-growing toenails. Yet we still insist on wearing crippling shoes and cutting our toenails in neat little rounded shapes!

Here's a guide to foot care with the accent on hygiene. Follow it and your feet will start to lead a meaningful, beautiful life.

1 Examine feet and lavish attention on them every bathtime. Check for corns, in-growing toenails, hard skin. Deal with the latter yourself or better still get a chiropodist to give your feet the once-over two or three times a year.

2 Cut toenails once a week, straight across to help prevent in-growth at the sides. It's amazing how many people forget to cut toenails, waiting until their shoes feel too tight before taking the plunge. Use sharp nail scissors or clippers; don't hack away with dressmakers' shears. Use a cuticle remover to deal with the bits of skin which seem to cling more lovingly to toenails than they do to fingernails. Dig out dirt trapped under the nail and down the sides of toes with a clean orange stick with the tip wrapped in a little cotton wool and dipped in cuticle remover. Paddle your toes in warm water first if you've been wearing open-toed shoes and the dirt is really thick.

3 Smooth feet with lavish dollops of body lotion or massage cream (try baby lotion) rubbed well in (but don't leave any sticky residue between the toes). Watch out for dark stubble around the ankle bones or on the big toe when de-fuzzing legs. Whisk it away regularly with a razor or depilatory cream. If you've got exceptionally hairy big toes then you can bleach them with a mild solution of peroxide. Do a skin-test on the inside of your arm first or have the hairs removed by waxing or electrolysis.

4 Beautify toes with polish . . . try the combined manicure and pedicure on page 93. When the polish gets chipped, apply another coat on top, but limit yourself to five coats before you start again.

5 Freshen feet (especially in hot weather) with regular use of a deodorizing foot spray or talc. The eccrine glands which produce perspiration are most active on the soles of the feet and palms of the hand. Hot, sticky hands get washed fairly often – feet don't. Foot odour seems to be a hereditary thing, but it is certainly aggravated by wearing nylon tights, nylon socks and synthetic-lined shoes. All three trap sweat and cause bacteria to multiply which can then lead to infection as well as a nasty smell. Choose leather shoes or canvas sneakers, and cotton or woollen socks. Wash tights and stockings daily and don't wear them at all in the sun. Men can buy socks with a built-in deodorant or charcoal liners for their shoes, but for some these devices are just another excuse for not washing their feet. Bully a beautiful but smelly-footed man with fragrant gifts: ripe Camembert or goats' milk cheeses ... he'll get the message eventually. Toes and feet like the feel of tingling cold water. Dabble tired feet in cold water laced with vinegar, *not* boiling mustard baths which will cause redness and remove the natural oils which keep feet smooth.

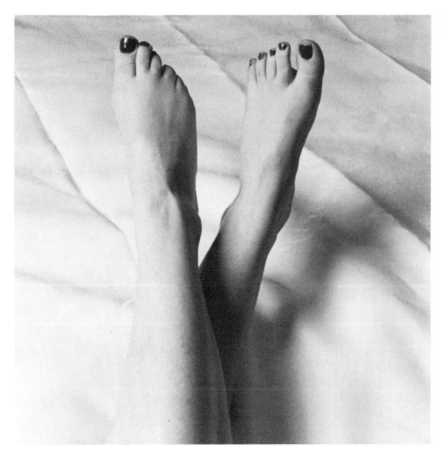

It may be corny, but if your feet hurt, it shows – on your face.

6 Strengthen feet and ankles with excercise. If you adore the highest possible heels, then your ankles will need strengthening. Try these effective exercises:

Sit on a chair, legs straight out in front. Point toes to ceiling then straight ahead, alternately. Now rotate feet clockwise, then anti-clockwise.

Drop a pencil on the floor and try to pick it up using bare toes.

Standing straight, rise up on tiptoe, hold the position briefly, then lower. Repeat rapidly, then try doing it with one foot at a time.

7 Walk barefoot as much as possible in the house if you have smooth flooring or carpet. Avoid soft carpet slippers – arches need good leather soles under them, not fluffy mules. Keep a comfy, well-made pair at home to change into after a day in fashionable shoes or boots. Try to shop around for shoes which are comfortable, wide-toed and well-supporting. Cramped toes invariably fight back by producing deformed nails or by dropping them off altogether. As nails take around a year to grow again, this can be a disaster if you want to have pretty feet in the bedroom and on the beach. It is also very painful! Make sure boots don't cramp calves and cut off the blood supply to your feet – you'll know all about it as your toes will go to sleep and attract chilblains.

Common foot nasties

Blisters are caused by pressure from shoes and boots. Leave off offending footgear and dab blister with surgical spirit.

Corns are caused by pressure and can be particularly painful when they are the soft type between the toes where infection is likely. The callous is a flat kind of corn usually on the ball of the foot. All three types need expert attention, not home treatment.

Verrucae are on the increase since the keep fit craze started. They are caused by a fungus infection found in gyms, swimming pools and jogging clubs, and produce a brownish, spotty sore. Avoid spreading them by contact, and see a specialist.

Athlete's foot is also on the increase and it too is a fungus infection, aggravated by woolly socks and soft shoes. Frankly, forget the trendy jogging until it clears up, otherwise you'll be in trouble.

In-growing toenails are caused by bad trimming and/or pressure. See a chiropodist for advice and treatment.

Bunions are misaligned joints which become swollen and tender. They can be cut out by surgery.

Walking on air? Good – bet your face looks a lot prettier too!

11 What about the Workers?

Indoors If you work in an office, school, light industrial factory or hospital you have nearly as many beauty hazards to face every day as an outdoor type. Central heating, air conditioning, dirt, dust and carbon paper are all potential problems. Then there's the journey to and from your work-place through torrential rain via dusty tube-trains, crowded buses and lead-laden traffic fumes. Here's how to cope:

Make-up and hair It's best to put on the full works at home, even though you may need to repair the ravages when you arrive. Start with moisturizer, top with a non-greasy liquid foundation in a pale colour (hot transport and a heated office will make you look rosy) with tawny blusher.

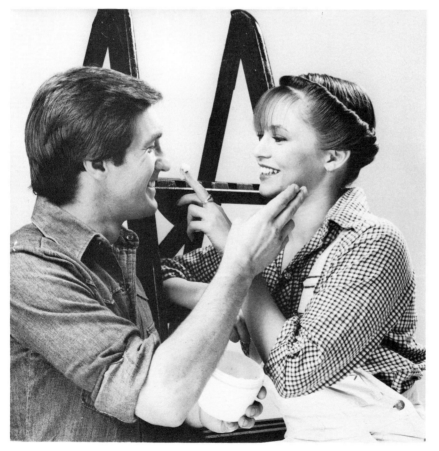

Everyone who does a tough job – male or female – needs to protect their skin. If you work outdoors, be specially careful about moisturizing hands as well as face.

Outline lips with a pencil to stop 'running' and fill in with a lipstick. If the morning looks wet and windy from your bedroom window, tuck your hair into a hat or roll into a pleat for the journey, brushing out when you arrive. A perm will actually improve in the rain. Long hair can be plaited and pinned on top for a peasant look which brushes out into pre-Raphaelite waves when you arrive. Keep powder, cleansing pads, foundation and a small spray of mineral water in your office desk to refresh your make-up at lunchtime or in the evening.

Hands and nails Typing, drawing, writing – they are all filthy jobs. Keep your own mild soap for frequent hand-washing, plus hand cream in your drawer. The old cliché about secretaries filing their nails all day needn't be true if you keep nails shortish, oval and use basecoat, plus two or three coats of toughened nail enamel to help prevent accidents. Then, instead of filing your nails in boring moments, you can spend your time plotting how to take over the boss's job.

Freshness If you've ever been on the receiving end of a whiff of BO from a colleague, you'll know how nasty it can be. Central heating makes everyone hot and bothered, and if you're working in a tense atmosphere with lots of panics and power struggles then nervous perspiration starts building up under even the coolest armpits. The nervous type is smellier than the hot-and-bothered type of perspiration. The eccrine glands secrete a milky fluid to which odour-producing bacteria are rapidly attached; the apocrine glands, responsible for the hot-and-bothered feeling, secrete a clear, odourless fluid. Together, these fluids attract bacteria like crazy! So, shower or bath in the morning and use a roll-on deodorant (more efficient and cheaper than the aerosol kind) under your arms. Keep another roll-on deodorant in your desk, wear cotton next to your skin, and count ten before you blow up in a crisis! Bad breath is another office plague – endless cups of coffee produce a musky, unpleasant smell, as do garlic-laden lunches, pub food and drink, and surreptitious sips of gin when things get tough.

Office equipment check list Toothbrush and toothpaste, mouthwash or mouth freshener, your favourite perfume (in an aerosol spray for speed and economy – they also prevent nasty spills over work), and spare stockings or tights.

Exercises for office workers

The twist This yoga position is complicated – but it's perfect for ironing out the aches and pains of a body that's been contorted over a cramped office desk all day.

Sit on the floor, both legs outstretched, hands by your sides. Cross your left leg over your right leg and place your left hand flat on the floor, as in the photograph. With your right hand grip the outside of your right leg,

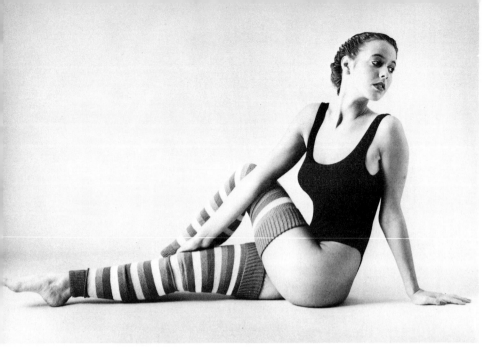

The twist.

then slowly twist to your left and look over your left shoulder. You'll feel your spine working and your shoulders and back feel more supple and strong.

Turn back to the front and repeat. Now repeat twice with the right leg crossed over the left and looking over your right shoulder.

The side bend This will keep your tum and waistline trim, despite those office snacks and endless cups of coffee; it will also relax the neck and shoulders.

Sit cross-legged on the floor and place your hands behind your neck. Slowly bend over to the right, keeping your tum tucked in. Straighten up, then bend to the left. Straighten up, then lean forward. Straighten up once more, and repeat the whole sequence ten times.

Outdoors If you're a lorry-driver, brickie, plumber's mate, heavy industry factory worker, mum with under-school-age children, stable lad, gas fitter – then you have very special beauty problems. The elements play havoc with skin, hair and nails, speeding up the ageing process, as well as contributing to immediate 'nasties' like dryness, soreness and split ends. Materials such as cement, axle grease, nappy cleanser, manure, etc., can cause allergic reactions, so wearing adequate protective clothing is a vital part of the job. There is also the problem of cleansing skin, hair and face every day *without* drying out the natural oils.

Here's a guide to coping with beauty care under these very special circumstances:

Skin You can always tell how old a male construction worker is – look at his face, make a guess, then *subtract* ten years. Women who face the

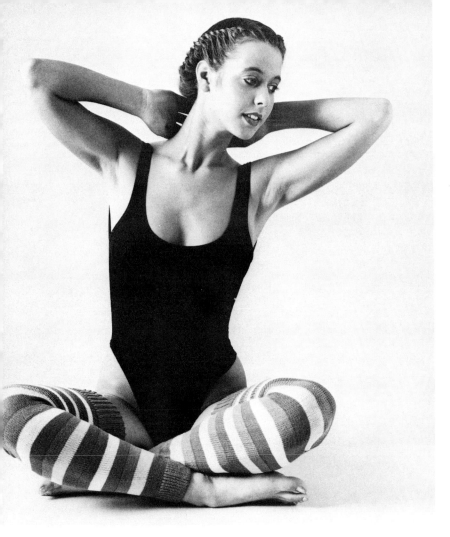

The side bend.

elements at work each day do have the protection of moisturizer and make-up which helps soften the skin. But both sexes should use a protect-tive colourless base each morning, and a softening cream at night. This will help prevent industrial dirt and fumes from leaping into your pores. Girls should top this with a fluid make-up and powder. In summer use a sun-screen on your face with a high protective factor even if you normally tan easily (three seasons 'on the job' will give you a leathery face very quickly), and a lower factor cream on the rest of the exposed skin areas. You'll sweat on the job, so wear natural fibre clothing to allow perspira-tion to evaporate naturally from your body, otherwise the sweat build-up will cause spots and blackheads on your back, chest or even bottom (people who drive for a living are particularly prone to problems in this area). Wear cotton pants, bra, and vest, topped with a T-shirt, shirt and woollen sweater or cotton overalls. Non-porous safety overalls are some-times regulation wear – take a cool bath after work and wash all over with a bland soap (no harsh detergent bubble bath) and then use body lotion or oil. This bathing technique applies to all outdoor workers; *don't* be tempted to soak for hours in a hot, soapy bath, however much elbow-grease you've used during the day. It will dry your skin and produce redness and soreness next day. *Do* add oil or a tablespoonful of cider vinegar to the water to soften it. At night, use anti-wrinkle cream on the eye area and 'concentration' lines: forehead, brow and the corners of the mouth.

Hair If a safety helmet is vital for your job, then wear it all the time. Tuck long hair inside, or fasten on top with a covered elastic band to prevent splitting. For outdoor work, shorter hair or a long hair-do, caught up in a pony tail or 'bunches', is best. Or, try the fashionable rolled or plaited look: make a side or middle parting, and roll the ends from the parting towards the crown of your hair, right around the head, fastening with hair pins or grips. If your hair is very long, tie a scarf around your head first, and roll your hair into that – like the land army girls of the 'forties. This style looks good with bright lipstick and blusher, and when it's unrolled the hair is prettily fluffed out. The French pleat of the 'fifties is also high fashion now and practical too: See page 41 for how to do it. A wash and wear perm is also practical (for both sexes) but needs weekly conditioning to prevent split ends, especially if it's coloured or highlighted. Most colours will 'lift' if you work outdoors, so it's most practical to stick to your natural shade, or to have the colour as near to that shade as possible, perhaps using a rinse or semi-permanent colourant to add sheen and tone. Highlights stand up to weather very well, as do 'lowlights' – these are coloured streaks put into the hair using a colourant rather than a bleaching agent; this can be a costly process.

If you must wash your hair every day, use just *one* application of shampoo and choose a *mild* shampoo (baby shampoo or a special shampoo for frequent washing such as Elsève Frequence by L'Oréal) with a conditioning rinse once or twice a week. A good conditioner for dry hair is coconut oil. Apply thickly, wrap hair in a hot towel and leave for one hour before shampooing. Have your hair trimmed regularly (or do this yourself – see page 36) to remove split ends and treat yourself to a cut and restyle when necessary.

Nails and hands Keep nails shortish, filed into an oval shape, and protect them with extra-tough nail enamel in a neutral or pinkish shade which doesn't look too nasty when chipped. Nourish nails with a protein conditioning cream and take time out for regular cleansing and manicure. If you're in a really dirty job, wear gloves. This is particularly important for men as dirty, calloused hands can be a real turn-off to the women in your life. If it's practical to do so, use a barrier cream: one teaspoon of Fuller's Earth, one teaspoon almond oil and one egg yolk is an effective mixture. But, in some cases, barrier creams could be dangerous as they might make

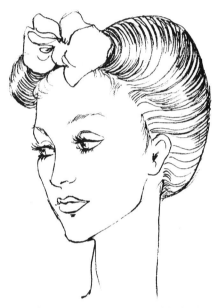

The 'forties roll is a practical hair-do for girls working in industry or in the open air. A scarf is tied round the head *over* the hair, then the hair is rolled up and tucked into the scarf. After work the hair can be brushed out into soft curls.

your hands slip at the wrong moment. In that case, top up conditioning treatment with a good hand cream at the end of your working day. Avoid drying soaps, washing up liquids and harsh chemicals. Dermatitis can be caused by any number of chemicals – if you have a problem, then consult your doctor immediately.

Eyes Wear safety glasses if it's a necessary part of your job – the British Safety Council say that men are more vain about not wearing glasses than women, and the further north you go, the more vain they are! If you wear eye make-up on the job make sure it's the hypo-allergenic kind; don't rub your eyes with dirty fingers, *ever*. Don't use waterproof mascaras as these are tough to remove and could cause eye irritation. Your best choice is a simple water-based block mascara or wand, plus cream or powder shadow and eyeliner above the lashes. Kohl liner worn around the rim of the eye is a waste of time as the wind and weather will quickly make the kohl run into your eyes. If your eyes hurt, bathe them with a solution of cold tea, or try compresses of cotton wool soaked in witch-hazel or slices of cucumber over each eye. On an outdoor job, good sunglasses can help prevent glare and wind irritating your eyes; invest in a pair with polarized lenses. Photochromic lenses (the kind that grow darker as natural light becomes more intense) are not recommended for drivers as they can be dangerous if you drive into a dark tunnel and then come out into strong sunlight (or vice versa). Have a regular eye check-up; a recent survey revealed that one-third of all workers either need *new* specs or need specs and don't realize it!

Lips and cheeks Carry an anti-chap stick in your overalls or jeans, and stroke it on to your lips when needed. If lipstick is practical, wear it, choosing a creamy formula containing lip balm and conditioning ingredients. You'll need to pencil in an outline before applying lipstick to prevent 'bleeding', blot lipstick then re-apply for a long-lasting effect. Don't bother with gloss: it will reduce the 'staying power' of your lipstick. If you have fine skin, beware of red veins and broken capilliaries in your cheeks. You need a good moisturizer and make-up to cover them up, and protect them. If you work inside, wear a powder blusher as a creamy one will attract dirt particles from the factory floor. Men with the same problem should cover red vein areas with a rich cream and perhaps use a 'cover stick' to protect the area during outdoor work.

Diet Hard work makes you *ravenous* but the calories taken in are often *not* expended in terms of physical work. In a tough, manual job you need 3,000 calories (male) or 2,500 calories (female), less if you are overweight. Beware of the pub or canteen lunch: beer or short drinks with sandwiches pile on the calories, with less protein than you really need for work output and staying power. So, start the day with a cooked breakfast of eggs, bacon, orange juice and wholemeal toast and honey *or* a quickie cold breakfast of ham or cheese with bread and honey or Marmite. If you have five minutes flat before catching the 5 am bus, whizz up a healthy high-protein drink: yogurt, orange juice, one egg, nutmeg and one spoonful honey. Take a packed lunch for economy and health: salad, cold ham or chicken, fresh fruit and hot home-made vegetable soup, natural fruit juice or milk to drink. If you have to eat a canteen lunch, choose a salad or simple meat or fish dish with vegetables, and fruit salad or yogurt

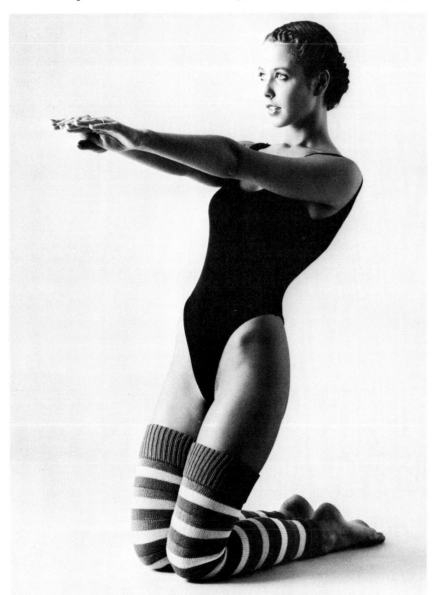

Keep your movements slow and graceful while doing the swan exercise ...

to follow. Remember that canteen vegetables have to be kept hot, destroying much of the important Vitamin C, so top up with extra fruit and vegetables when you are at home.

Exercises for exhausted bodies If your work is making your limbs creak and groan, try these easy yoga exercises which will help sort out those twinges:
The swan Kneel on the floor, then sit back on your heels. Raise your arms

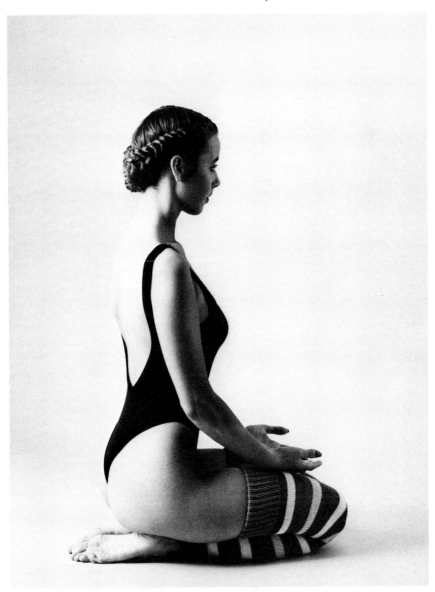

. . . and you will calm your mind as well as your body.

in the air and bring them down slowly in front of you, bending forward until your forehead touches the floor. Feel your neck stretching a bit. Now raise yourself up and forward into the 'all fours' position. Slide your hands forward, lower your pelvis and stretch upwards with your neck, head well back. Then sit back on your heels, arms stretched forward, head down. Relax by bringing your arms back by your sides. Repeat five times. *The cat* Start in the same position as above, and lean forward to the 'all fours' position. Hollow your back, then arch it, lowering your head. Repeat ten times, slowly.

Spoil yourself One night a week, allow yourself a luxurious beauty farm night at home to help counteract the effects of honest toil. Massage warmed olive oil into hands and feet, then take a comfortably hot bath scented with perfumed oils. A shampoo and blow-dry followed by the combined manicure and pedicure on page 93 will make you feel a different person. Afterwards, pamper yourself with a thorough massage all over to rub away the strain and tension of the day.

The cat.

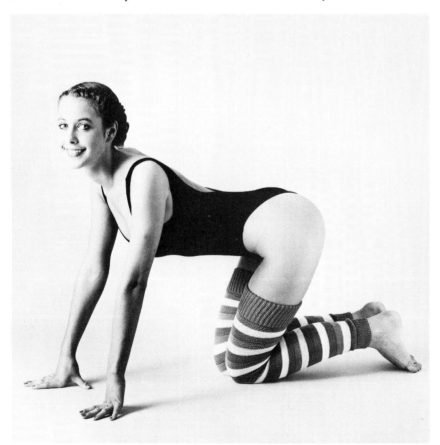

The step-by-step massage

You need a warm room with sufficient space to lie down; a towel; body lotion; tissues.

1 Lie on your back and relax for a minute. Pour a little lotion on your tummy and rub it in with circular movements.

2 Roll over. Press your fingertips on either side of your spine and rub gently. Bring your hands above shoulder level and rub shoulder blades, neck and shoulders in stroking movements.

3 Sit up slowly, take some more lotion and knead and press your legs. Work from the thighs towards the knees, then back again. Now do from the knees down to the ankles and back again.

4 Still sitting, press the tips of your thumbs either side of your spine. Press for a few seconds, relax and move your thumbs up about an inch. Repeat, working up as far as you can.

5 Stand up and knead and pinch your buttocks!

6 Finally, sit on a chair (cover it with your towel, as you're bound to be very oily indeed by this time) and work body lotion into your feet. The easiest way to do this is to rest one foot on the opposite thigh (like a modified 'half lotus' yoga position) and work really hard with fingers and thumbs all over the sole of your foot and between your toes. Repeat with the other foot.

7 Now blot off the surplus oil, put on a bathrobe and rest for at least an hour or as long as you can.

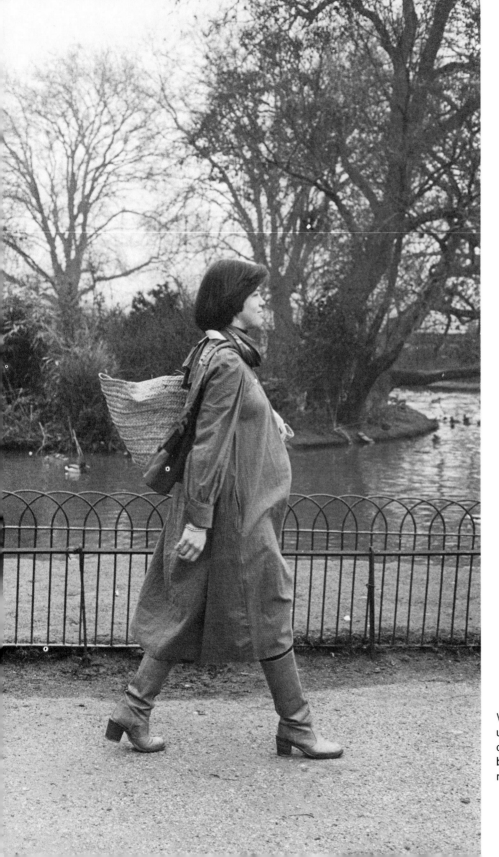

With your doctor's approval, keep up daily walks right to the very end of your pregnancy — if you are fit before the birth you will recover more quickly.

12 Beauty for Mums-to-be

Pale, baggy-eyed, nauseous, irritable – you can always tell when a girl's pregnant by the state of health of her man! Seriously, during the first three months, *both* halves of a child-rearing partnership need extra health and beauty care. Later you will both need just one thing – *sleep*!

For her Frantic hormonal activity produces problems like spots, lank hair, insomnia, exhaustion, nausea. Start the day with tea and dry toast or a biscuit in bed, camouflage your facial imperfections with extra make-up care, keep hair shortish and wash it frequently. Don't leap straight into huge maternity dresses – you'll get very bored indeed later. Instead, let out trouser and skirt waistbands and use the 'layered' look to flatter your pudding shape as much as possible. Start lubricating tummy, breasts, bottom and thighs with baby oil or a special cream to help prevent stretch marks. Latest nutritional thinking is that inadequate zinc during pregnancy may be partly responsible for these marks so step up seafood and fresh vegetables if you can. Drink that extra pinta or take calcium tablets to help build healthy bones for your babe, eat oily fish (which contains Vitamin D – essential for the baby, too) such as mackerel and sardines, liver and lots of fresh fruit and vegetables. Ruthlessly cut out fatteners like sweets, cakes and chocolates. If you are too sick to even *think* about liver or mackerel, let your doctor know so additional vitamins in the form of pills can be prescribed – otherwise the baby will take them from you, leaving you feeling extra weak and watery after the birth.

For him Combat that haggard, worried look with extra exercise and anti-stress routines like walking, making love and going to bed early (sex *won't* hurt the baby – unless your lady's doctor has specifically told her to stop having intercourse, it's safe to continue). Nausea and sympathetic twinges are natural, and should be treated with a simple, non-spicy diet and lots of love!

The final six months Pregnant ladies almost always find that things improve dramatically as the pregnancy proceeds. Hair becomes beautifully thick and glossy, skin almost translucent and vitality seems limitless. Play up your good looks with fabulous make-up and pretty clothes. Get plenty of exercise – walking and swimming are best. Wear medium-heeled shoes or boots at work to give your legs a fighting chance of supporting your extra bulk comfortably, and put your feet up for half an hour at the end of the working day. Continue with a super diet – remember that the babe is a selfish little creature who will drain your body of essential nutrients given half a chance. If you feel hot and bothered, take long cool baths and wear only natural cotton or light wool clothes.

This is often a girl's only chance of flaunting a sexy cleavage – enjoy it. *Do watch your weight.* Aim for a weight-gain of 22 lbs. Extra won't give you a bigger, healthier baby or make you a more successful breast-feeder. (In fact, a recent study in Cambridge showed that mums who were fatter in pregnancy were *less* successful.) It *will* make you more susceptible to high blood-pressure, toxaemia and birth complications.

If you have a demanding job, rest at lunchtime, but keep working as long as you feel up to it.

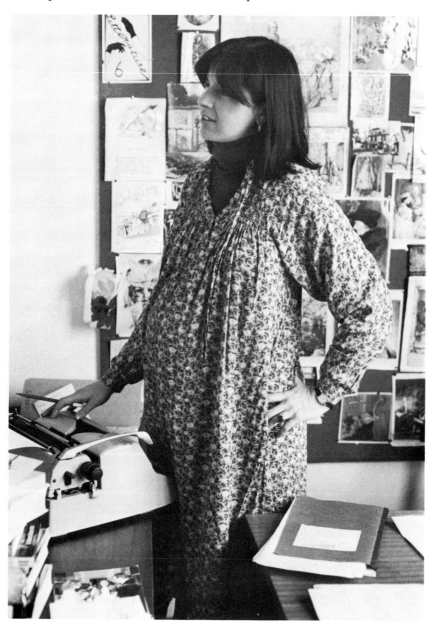

At this stage it makes sense to go along to your local ante-natal classes regularly or to attend a course run by an organization such as the National Childbirth Trust. These classes are a beauty treatment in themselves as well as highly informative and helpful – all that deep breathing makes you feel just great. If you're fit and well, avoid the temptation of stopping work too early – you'll get fat and fed up at home. When I had my first son, I worked up until Christmas Eve and produced him in one-and-a-half hours on the day after Boxing Day. When I had my second, I foolishly decided to work at home for the last three weeks of the pregnancy – result: extra weight-gain, and a very sluggish babe. Eventually, he was induced and appeared very rapidly indeed (two hours!), but I became extremely bored and boring during those weeks at home. Nature intended us to keep active . . . not to sit knitting tiny garments, nibbling chocolates and being fussed over!

Your B-Day beauty gear Most hospitals give you a check list of items to tuck in your suitcase ready for the big day – including such glamorous things as cotton nursing bras and extra large sanitary towels. Also essential: a quarter bottle of champagne tucked into your spongebag, a *huge* bottle of your favourite perfume, nail varnish, de-fuzzing cream, at least four pretty nightdresses (front opening, long sleeves), a sensational long housecoat, combs, ribbons, and slides for your hair, heated rollers, hair-dryer and shampoo plus conditioner. Hospitals usually wake up new mums at around 6 am. You feed your babe and then there's a long lull before breakfast – use it for nail polish renewing, hair-washing, etc. Don't miss out on the period in your life when there's actually time to kill by being badly equipped.

Post-natal beauty After all that get-up-and-glow during pregnancy, it's a blow to feel lumpy, depressed and panicky afterwards. First, remember that your hair is quite likely to drop out in handfuls – it *will* grow again, but meantime don't make things worse by indulging in panic measures like a harsh perm or a radical colour change – your body is not yet up to such strains, and the results are bound to be disappointing. Concentrate instead on getting your figure in trim: your body will quickly get back into shape if you do the right exercises (*see below*) and you will feel a lot better if you eat correctly. You need an extra 500 calories a day, plus fluids, if you're breast-feeding (even then, you will *lose* weight more quickly than non-breast-feeding mums) and make sure it's in the form of fresh produce: milk, meat and fish, plus stout if you like it. Otherwise, keep to 1,500 calories a day, but cut out all nasties like sweets, sugary puds and stodgy foods. Wholewheat bread is essential – two to three slices a day – to help supply the B vitamins you need to combat stress and tiredness. For the same reason, liver is worth getting to love just now – try it curried. Beautywise, take time out for a facial, hair-cut or massage at some time during the first two weeks after the birth (take the babe with you). Get into the habit of putting on make-up and doing your hair after the early morning feed, otherwise you could find yourself still in your housecoat at 4 pm. If you go straight back to work, try to combine work with breast-feeding at least for a few weeks. If you have a reasonable employer who'll let you start late and finish early, there is no reason why your baby should object to a combination of bottle and breast, and your body will soon adapt to producing milk at the right time of day. Breast-feeding is very relaxing at the end of a busy working day – better than two gin-and-tonics and twice as rewarding. A breast-pump and sterilized bottle is a handy extra in your office desk if you are in the kind of job where meetings and crises always crop up at 5 pm.

You will probably find that your skin becomes blotchy, your nails brittle and your teeth look a bit dingy soon after the birth. Use a good night cream and covering make-up, trim nails shortish and wear a strengthened nail polish. Cash in on *free* dentistry for a check up and scale and polish session. It really does take your body a full year to recover from childbirth, so don't expect miracles. But be a bit selfish too – limit socializing to the things you really want to do, and let others entertain you for a change. New babies are adaptable little souls – later, you won't be able to take them to parties in a carrycot, so it's worth making the effort while you can. It's also excellent for your looks and morale to dress up, paint your toenails and flirt!

The best ever post-natal exercise plan

This series of exercises was devised by a hospital physiotherapist to help new mums get back their pre-pregnancy figures and (most important) to tone up the pelvic and vaginal muscles that stretch to accommodate the baby as it passes through the birth canal. If you want a super post-baby figure and a good sex life, practise these every day for six months. They start on the first day after the birth, so if there are complications you must obviously check with your doctor.

Start all the exercises with six to eight movements, then gradually increase. The first day's exercises should be repeated on the second day, the first and second day's on the third day, and so on until all the exercises are repeated every day. They are super for a new dad's figure as well as a new mum, and great fun for young children. All lying down movements are fine on a fairly firm bed or a carpeted floor.

B-Day plus one
1 Lie on the bed with knees bent, and breathe in and out rhythmically and evenly.
2 Lie with legs straight and rotate feet and ankle to the left and right. Now tighten and relax knee muscles.

B-Day plus two

1 Lie with knees bent and tighten abdominal muscles and buttocks, pressing the natural hollow out of your back.

2 Lie with legs crossed at the ankles and contract pelvic floor muscles (these are the muscles that hold your vaginal area in place; to find them, 'spend a penny' then stop in mid-flow – these are your pelvic floor muscles!)

B-Day plus three

1 Lie with your hands on your hips. Draw up one hip, and push down with the other hip. Repeat the opposite way round.

2 Lie with knees bent, raise your head and left arm so that the left hand touches the right knee. Repeat with right arm and left knee.

3 Stand against a wall. Push the small of your back against the wall, pull in tummy and stand 'tall' to correct posture. Shoulders should be straight, bottom tucked in, knees braced, chin in and head up.

B-Day plus four

1 Lie down, raise your right leg and swing it over to the left. Raise to straight position, then lower. Repeat with the other leg.

2 Kneel on all fours, arch back slowly, then hollow it.

B-Day plus five

1 Lie down, legs together. Raise right hand to touch left ankle. Repeat with opposite arm and leg.

2 Stand against wall with trunk dropped loosely downwards. Uncurl slowly, feeling almost every vertebra touching the wall until you're standing up straight.

B-Day plus six

1 Kneel on all fours, raise right knee to touch your nose, stretch your leg slowly backwards and lower it. Repeat with the other leg.

2 Lie on your back, legs together. Raise your knees to tummy-level, circle them once, then return to first position.

13 A Climate for Beauty

Like local wine, people sometimes just don't travel well. We're all greatly influenced by our climate and surroundings. Our bodies are programmed by genetic and environmental factors to behave well under certain conditions; change those conditions and confusion sets in.

So, if you're off on a trip to the tropics, a jumbo flight to another continent or a holiday in the sun, it just isn't enough to pack your heated rollers and a tube of suntan cream. If you want to stay looking and feeling good, get clued-up on how you can expect your body to react to all the changes which are likely . . . from food and drink to humidity.

Skin The acid mantle which covers and protects your skin varies slightly depending on where you live, so a journey to a spot that's miles away is bound to affect you, even if the spot concerned is in this country. If you're going somewhere hot, follow the chart on page 79 for sun protection – even if it's a business trip and you don't intend to spend hours baking on the beach. Wherever you're going, consider first the kind of food you'll be eating when you arrive.

If the food is greasier than you're used to (Southern Europe, Northern England, North Africa), the pores of your skin will excrete more sebum than usual. Unless you have a very dry skin normally, it's best to pack light water-based lotions, instead of gooey creams. If your skin is sensitive, oily sun lotion on top of the extra oil coming from your pores could cause a fry-up, so use a product with a high sun-protection factor.

Spicy additions to the menu may trigger off skin reactions too. Sheep's eyeballs in spicy sauce and black pudding may increase the irritant secretions from your pores on to your skin . . . the same goes for exotic rum punches! You need to be extra scrupulous about cleansing: two goes with a light cleanser and clean cotton wool, followed up with a non-alcoholic tonic lotion. If the country is very hot, there's an extra problem: sweat. People who live in the tropics have more sweat glands per square centimetre than Northern Europeans or Americans (about 558.9 glands per square centimetre for Caucasians, 738.2 glands per square centimetre for Asians and Africans). So, when we visit a sultry spot our poor glands have to cope with pumping out extra sweat, plus the irritant secretions contained in it. This causes the open-pored leathery look that's a characteristic of cold-climate mortals who travel to hot spots frequently.

If your trip means less greasy food and more exposure to cold air (Scandinavia, Northern Canada), then pack some richer skin-food and be prepared for dry skin patches which will need a greasier make-up and soothing creams. Your lips will need special treatment too.

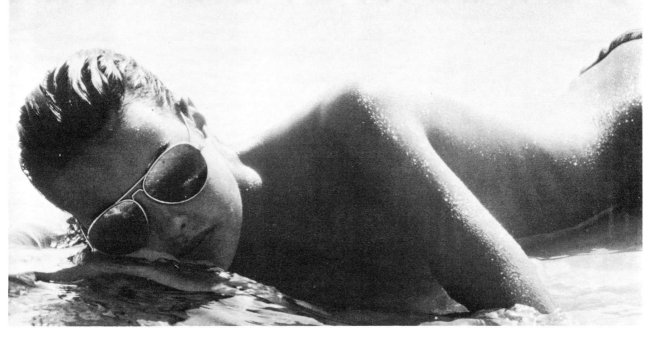

Hotel heating and air-conditioning are also big skin hazards. For some reason, hoteliers love bringing guests down to freezing level or up to boiling point in the middle of the night. If your skin gets icy blasts at night after a day in the sun it will feel tight and sore. If you're in the north, or the United States in winter, and the heat is well and truly on, sleep with nothing on your face – face creams would be washed away with the perspiration. Instead, cleanse thoroughly and apply rich moisturizer before you venture outside into the cold.

Hair Expect your hair to play up on your travels and you'll probably be agreeably surprised at how well it behaves! Anyway, do be prepared for the worst, especially if you go to a hot, humid country. The only kind of hair-do to have when you're travelling is a wash-and-wear perm which simply needs combing through with your fingers, *or* a simple straightish style which you can wash and set in your hotel room with a few rollers or a hair-dryer and brush. Have colours or perms done before you go. If it's a long trip, ask your hairdresser to write down your colour formula for you – at least that will give you a starting point for foreign hairdressers (it's a comforting thought that products from Clairol, Wella and Schwarzkopf are available almost everywhere in the world these days). Your natural pigment is likely to be 'thrown' by your change of diet (the quality and type of protein, animal or vegetable, which you consume affects the colour and condition of your hair) and strong sunlight – so you may well need to re-think your colour completely if you're staying for a long time. Keep tinted hair covered in strong sunlight, watch for signs of dryness and use a conditioner every time you wash it. Don't overdo the roller-setting. On holiday, a tan will help you get away with a much more casual look, so concentrate on good condition rather than a complicated style.

Don't forget that suntan lotions wash off in the sea, so if you want to build up an even, healthy tan, apply more the minute you have dried off.

Body Wear cotton clothes to allow perspiration to evaporate naturally in hot countries, and take your lead from the natives in cold countries; if everyone sports a cotton vest and layers of wool, do the same. Watch out for fluid retention problems – these often occur if you travel to very hot countries . . . although you perspire so much, the body seems to store up fluid in odd places: ankles, tummy and thighs. Alcohol definitely makes this problem worse, so stick to mineral water if you can. Avoid using anti-perspirant products *ad lib* in hot countries . . . shower two or three times a day instead.

Putting on weight will obviously be a problem if you're off on holiday or on a business trip to hospitable parts of the world. The only way to cope is to give yourself a 5 lb ceiling. When you have reached it, hold back for a day or two.

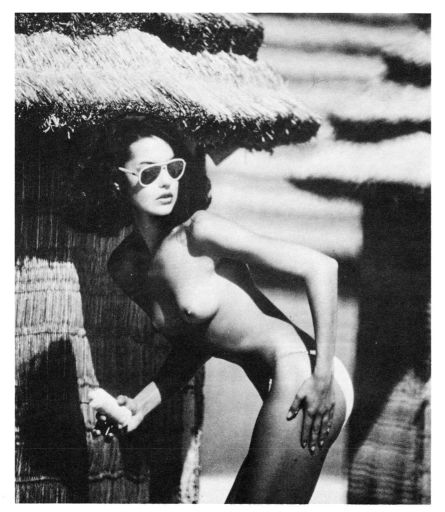

Give special attention to parts of your body that don't often see the light!

Your suntan guide Start to prepare your body for sun exposure *before* you go on holiday. Increase your intake of Vitamin A (in carrots, apricots, butter, eggs) since this vitamin is depleted by the sun, and without it the risk of burning is increased. Prepare your skin by taking warm baths with baby oil (one teaspoon in the bath is adequate), and rubbing down your body with more baby oil or body lotion afterwards. Pay particular attention to skin areas which don't usually get much exposure to the elements and will certainly get some on holiday: chest (and breasts if you intend to go topless), tummy, back, neck, upper arms and legs. If you can, catch some watery northern sunshine by using a suntan preparation containing bergamot oil, which actually intensifies the sun's rays. Snatch a few hour-long sunbathing stints at weekends to start off your suntan.

There are now so many suntan preparations on the market that the choice can be bewildering. Many are marked with a factor number (which is supposed to be uniform throughout the various brands, but actually does vary a little in strength). Briefly, the higher the number the more protection you get from the dangerous ultra-violet rays. More explicitly, the factor number denotes the *time* you can stay in the sun. For instance, if you normally start going pink in ten minutes, by applying a lotion with factor number 2 you *double* the time – so you won't go pink until twenty minutes are up. With factor number 3, you *treble* the time, and so on.

This chart gives an at-a-glance guide to the factor numbers to go for, according to your destination and skin type:

Sun strength	**Your skin type**					
	Fair – burns easily		*Normal – burns but tans easily too*		*Dark – tans fast*	
	Not yet tanned	When you start to tan	Not yet tanned	When you start to tan	Not yet tanned	When you start to tan
Moderate (Northern Europe, Britain)	5	3	3	2	2	2
Strong (Central Europe, the Mediterranean)	7	5	5	3	3	2
Intense (Southern Europe, Middle East, North Africa and high altitudes)	7	7	7	5	7	5

NB All skin types need a high protective factor (7) on nipples, breasts and buttocks.

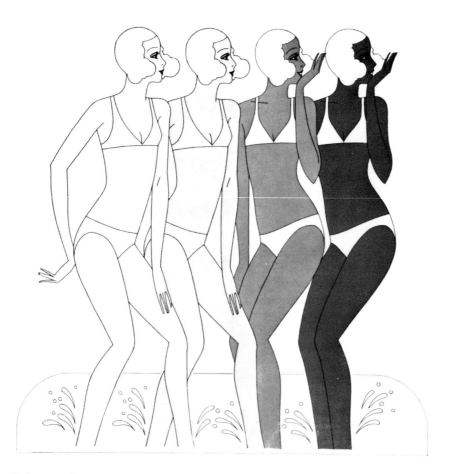

Fake tanning preparations These contain a substance which blends with the melanin in the skin to produce a brownish pigment. They are harmless, but should be applied with great care for an even and convincing result. First prepare the skin with all over body lotion, then rub in the fake tan with sweeping massage movements, concentrating on one area at a time so you don't forget where you've applied it. Blot dry absorbent areas like knees and elbows with tissue, and wash hands thoroughly. Use a fake tan to keep up a natural tan when you return home or before you go on holiday. It *won't* prevent your skin from burning, but it will make you less abandoned about rushing into the sun on your first few days – and that's when most harm is usually done.

What to do if you are burned If the soreness isn't too severe take a cold bath (no soap) and apply cool, wet compresses to the painful bits. However if you are blistered, feel sick or are in acute pain, see a doctor *immediately*. For very mild sun-reddening, cold tea or calomine lotion makes an effective cooling treament.

Pills and your tan If you are on the Pill, you may find that your skin is more sensitive to the sun, and tans more quickly. The Pill may also cause extra skin-sensitivity, as may other drugs – antibiotics, tranquillizers, sedatives or diuretics – so if you experience unusually violent sunburn or red patches and swelling, check your medical list. Externally applied substances such as perfume, cosmetics, skin tonics or even sun lotions sometimes trigger off a similar reaction.

Ageing and the sun There is absolutely no doubt that the sun dries and ages the skin. So, if you're over twenty-five don't expose your face to the sun day in, day out unless you want to look like a wrinkled prune at forty! Some cosmetic companies have produced anti-wrinkle creams which contain sun-creams and are specially designed for the sun . . . but these are protective, not preventative, so they won't help if you insist on frying!

14 On the Road

If you have to spend a lot of time in your car, it makes sense to be as comfortable as possible. First, check your car seat for comfort: car interiors are notoriously badly designed. For good posture, you should sit upright, with good vision over the wheel, legs comfortably stretched out to the pedals (*not* with your knees under your chin). You may well find that a cushion or light padding behind you, and a *cotton* covering on the seat itself is far more comfortable than sticky plastic-type seating. Shoes must be well-fitting and comfortable – keep a special pair in the car to change into, plus foot spray and talc for freshness. Sticky hands can be a problem too: talc and cologne are handy, tucked into the dashboard. Have your eyes tested: the ability to read a number plate at a distance of twenty-five yards does *not* indicate good eyesight. Clean your windscreen often to prevent eyestrain, and make sure your lights are well adjusted. On long journeys, take a rest whenever you feel 'off' or bored – don't wait until you're dead tired, that's when accidents happen. Expert Dr Keith Jolles recommends layby stops every two hours.

Make-up tends to go shiny in your car, so keep it light with a liquid foundation, blusher, lipstick and eye make-up only. Tie long hair back from your face with a pretty scarf or knot it on top, otherwise it could spoil your vision during a complicated manoeuvre: the fantasy girl who drives a white sports car with long hair flying all over the place is actually a terrible hazard. Don't wear long floaty scarves at the wheel either – Isadora Duncan, the dancer, did just that, and you remember what happened to *her*!

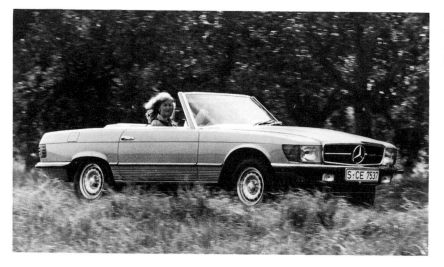

Step up moisturizing when you are on the road – even if you aren't in an open car your skin will quickly become dehydrated.

The worst beauty hazard for motorists is food. Motorway cafés tend to serve up stodgy meals, although there are usually some salads, fruit and yogurt available. Unfortunately, stodge *inside* your tum makes you feel stodgy *outside*, and it could be a danger. Lots of drinks can have an upsetting effect; being stuck in a traffic jam while you're aching to spend a penny is not a happy experience. Tea and coffee are only short-term stimulants: the best drink to take on a long journey is a flask containing the juice of two lemons with one tablespoon honey, topped up with boiling water. Sip this drink at each layby stop to boost your blood sugar level and make you feel bright and brilliant. Nibble fruit and cold meat for extra energy without sluggishness.

When you stop, do some exercises to help ease cramps and stop that 'long distance spread'.

Exercises at the wheel

1 Press hands against the wheel at the 'quarter to three' position, pushing your feet down on to the floor at the same time. Hold for a count of six, then relax. This helps trim and strengthen arms, bottom, bosom and thighs.
2 Clasp hands in front of your nose. Now look up and stretch arms upwards (hands still clasped). Lower hands behind your head, push elbows back. Hold briefly, raise arms, lower and relax. This helps relieve aching shoulder and back muscles.
3 Sit well back in your seat, fold your arms. Raise left knee, now rotate foot clockwise, then anticlockwise. Repeat with right knee and foot. Now point toes twenty times. This helps strengthen and relax tired feet and trim ankles which often get puffy in a warm car.
With your co-driver Do these relaxing exercises which are super on those long, long drives through France or down to the West Country:
4 Place your fingers on his scalp and move the skin in a circular motion – it feels delicious and will do his hair good as well as relax him!
5 Sitting behind him, massage his shoulder blades, then pull his elbows back fairly sharply. Repeat ten times.
6 Place your fingertips lightly over his eyelids, tickle them lightly, then bring fingertips outwards to the outer corner of his eyes. Repeat five times.

Now change gear – with *you* on the receiving end of these soothing exercises.

15 Beauty on a Shoe-string

When the bank balance is low and you can't afford to rush out and spend a fortune on a perm or a facial, you can still look a million dollars. By trial and error, I've found that there are lots of ways to cut corners and save money on beauty products.

Here are my top penny-pinching ideas:

1 Check through your existing make-up to find old products that suddenly look new, or could be used in a new way. For instance, last year's pink blusher could look wonderful as this year's eye shadow; two or three old lipsticks could be melted down to make a pot of new lipgloss (use empty eye-shadow cases to hold the brew which should be melted in a china dish over hot water).

2 Check the cheaper make-up ranges for small, inexpensive items to add instant appeal to your looks. Good names: Rimmel (always first with new colours, new products and wonderful value), Miners, Tu. Choose products which are versatile as well as new: rust eye shadow which doubles as blusher, one super plum pencil that looks good on eyes, mouth and cheek and happens to be the 'in' colour, a huge bottle of skin cream that's smashing for your body too.

3 Stretch out the lasting-power of existing favourite products so you don't have to spend money on more: cut circles of cotton or lint and 'sandwich' between eye make-up remover pads to double the value. Always apply water-based foundations with a water-soaked pad of cotton wool or a cosmetic sponge: the water dilutes the foundation slightly and makes it last much longer. (If liquid foundations dry out, you can usually add a little water to make them last until funds become available!)

4 Discover the versatility of baby products (and the baby prices): baby oil is good as an eye make-up remover, bath additive, body rub. Use baby lotion as a cleanser and moisturizer for the whole body. Baby powder is super as talc, face powder (brush off surplus – it gives a pale, pearly finish to your make-up) and dry shampoo in emergencies.

5 Make up your own inexpensive brews. My favourite home-made concoction is simply a bottle of corn oil with cider vinegar (two parts oil, one part vinegar) which is added to bath water and used as a hair conditioner and tanning lotion. Fuller's Earth is a cheap substance to buy from chemists and can be used with a variety of household products to make face-packs. Try mixing a dessertspoon of Fuller's Earth with an egg and a drop of olive oil for a nourishing face-mask. Lemons are versatile too: use lemon juice with yogurt or milk as a skin lotion (rub on, allow to dry, then rinse off with tepid water) for greasy skins: use lemon juice with beaten

egg white and a few drops of rose-water as a greasy skin mask; cut lemon in half and rub the inside peel on elbows to soften them and nails to strengthen them. Lemon is also a bleaching agent and will make blonde hair go lighter if stroked on to the hair while you sunbathe.

However poor you happen to be you'll look a rich lady if your hair is glossy and well-cut, your eyebrows well-shaped and your skin good. Save your pennies for a haircut, and concentrate on getting the condition right – pile it on top while you wait for that windfall!

There's also no time like no-cash time for going on a slimming diet. Ruthlessly cut out expensive cakes, sweets and alcohol, and concentrate on fruit, vegetables, fish or meat and cheaper dry white wine (lower in calories than expensive gin). Your figure will improve; so will your looks.

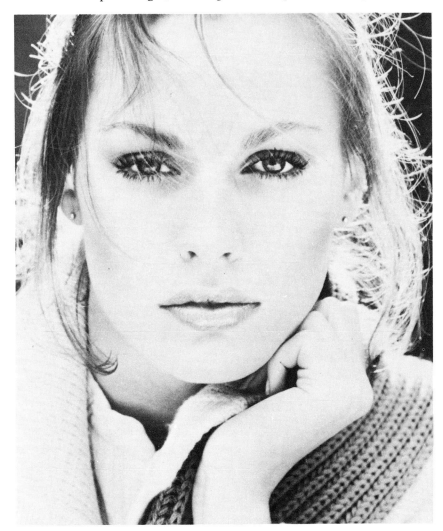

You *can* look great on a shoe-string! Walking to work will do wonders to your figure and complexion.

16 Beauty when you're Feeling Lavish

If you get a windfall at Christmas or on your birthday, then there are a number of good beauty investments to spend it on. *Don't* fritter the lot away on a miracle cream that might make you look better; spend it on treatments that *will* make you look better. There's nothing like a salon treatment to boost your morale. I recommend these:

Cathiodermie This is a deep-cleansing treatment invented in Paris but now widely available at salons in this country. It is based on a weak electric current transmitted via rollers and metal spheres used in conjunction with special cleansing gels on the face. Sounds horrific, but is in fact one of the most relaxing and beneficial treatments I know, especially when your skin is looking 'muddy' or jaded after a holiday or a long cold winter. Good for men too and certainly excellent for the acne-prone. Cost – from about £8, according to the salon and accompanying treatments. Addresses on page 104.

Aromatherapy Body or facial massage using essential oils geared to specific problems: tension, acne, dry skin, cellulite, even constipation. Treatment is based on methods developed in Paris (again!) by the late Marguerite Maury, a top beautician who travelled extensively in the Far East. All the oils smell delicious and you are literally soothed into ecstasy by the treatment! Recommended when you're run-down or just need pampering. Prepare to feel exalted and a bit sexy afterwards! Lots of salons now specialize in aromatherapy: addresses of the best ones are on page 105. Cost – about £6 plus, according to how much of you is massaged!

Paraffin wax treatment This is usually a treatment given in conjunction with a course of massage and exercise for slimming problems, but it is also a delicious experience if you have dry skin. You are cocooned in white paraffin wax which dries and makes your body sweat. At the same time the wax softens your skin beautifully. Some salons also use this treatment for hands (during a manicure), or feet. Cost – from about £3.50.

Day of beauty Many salons and health clubs now offer an inclusive all-day rate for girls who want to spend a full day pampering themselves and being pampered. The price will include such things as sauna, massage, exercising, facial and suntan treatments – from about £15. I particularly recommend a day spent at The Sanctuary in Covent Garden, London (full details on page 111) where £10 buys you a sumptuous day in beautiful surroundings – swimming, sunbathing on special treatment beds (no risk of burning and a natural, gradual tan) and use of hair-drying and setting facilities and gym. Bliss.

As well as the specialist treatments above, you could also spend your windfall on a good perm, leg-waxing (from about £6), or a make-up lesson

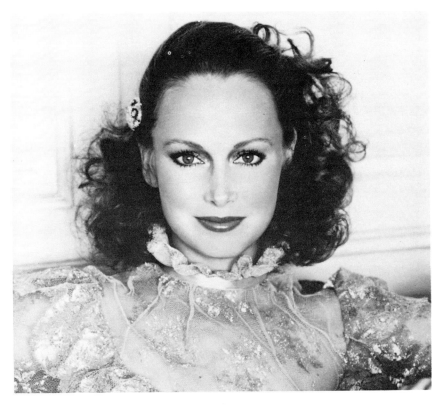

When the money comes rolling in, spend it on beauty treats to make you feel, and look, pampered.

at one of the salons on page 106. If you're in the *big* money you might like to invest in a course of beauty therapy, make-up or manicure – from £200 plus. Jobs are now more plentiful in the beauty industry for girls with the right qualifications, so the investment may well pay off with big returns.

A visit to a health farm (full list on page 110) could be a good idea if you feel very exhausted and overweight. But you must go to the hydro with the right attitude; be prepared to toe the line and co-operate with the regime imposed. It's not a good idea to go to a way-out cranky establishment if you adore three square meals a day and don't really need to diet. I recommend Champneys at Tring for the luxury classes, particularly for men as their no-nonsense medical approach is sensible and appeals to the male animal! If money is less abundantly available, I recommend Ragdale Hall in Leicestershire which is run by *Slimming Magazine* and is very sensible indeed about diet (you don't starve) but has some excellent beauty treatments too. It's best to go to a health farm alone or with a *very* dear companion or lover. No one looks their best in a functional dressing-gown, clutching a lettuce leaf, and some beautiful friendships have floundered under such circumstances. Arm yourself with books and be prepared to sleep a lot. The treatments, coupled with the low-calorie diet, are extremely exhausting.

17 Beauty in a Hurry

I once calculated that I wasted approximately two hours every year of my life just opening and closing eye-shadow packs looking for the shade I need every morning. A top make-up artist, Celia Hunter, put me right with an idea that's so simple it hurts: remove the little metal containers holding compressed powder shadow from the individual boxes and put the whole lot in one plastic or cardboard box (sponge-lined) together with a selection of suitable brushes. If all your make-up is similarly displayed in a knife drawer tucked into the top drawer of your dressing table, then you'll save hours of hunting time – you'll also save money, since refill packs are just as good as posh ones for this kind of organization. Save time too, by keeping the right tools for the job in the right spot for immediate use: eyebrow tweezers in the room with the best light, not necessarily the bedroom; hand cream in the kitchen; perfume beside your bed; nail polish hidden away in the sitting-room if you do your nails watching TV; moisturizer in the bathroom; tissues just about everywhere; slimming diet sheets in the kitchen; barrier cream in the garden shed.

You can also save hours by combining several beauty jobs at once: for example, sitting in the bath with hair conditioner on then showering *all over*; doing facial exercises while you clean your teeth; giving yourself a face-mask while defuzzing your legs (it gives you something to do while you're waiting for the depilatory lotion to work); soaking up body oil while you give yourself a naked manicure and pedicure; letting your hair dry naturally while you do exercises in the garden.

Get your morning routine running smoothly and quickly. After your shower, apply moisturizer in the bathroom so that it has time to sink in as you nip back to your bedroom; consult wardrobe, open make-up drawer (brilliantly laid out as above!) and decide on colours. Try the following thorough make-up routine, which is particularly handy when you're travelling or on holiday or otherwise don't want to lose a second.

Ten minute make-up

You need large rouge mop brush, cotton buds (for eye make-up and pencil 'smudging'), cotton wool, tissues, hairband, moisturizer or baby lotion, eyebrow brush and tweezers.
Cosmetics Foundation toned to skin, translucent powder, eyebrow pencil, water-based wand eye shadow in a neutral colour such as beige or peach, eye pencil and/or powder shadow, mascara, lip pencil, lipstick and gloss, powder shaders and blushers.

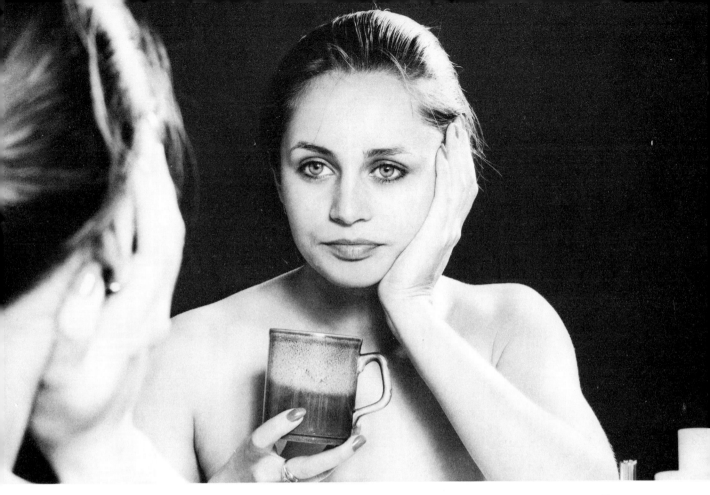

1 Fasten hair securely back from your face. Apply moisturizer in small dabs all over your face and smooth into your skin with gentle *upward* strokes, including the eye area.

2 Now apply your foundation, again with little dabs. Smooth in lightly with *downward* strokes: this is to follow the natural hair-growth and give a smooth look to your face. Make sure you apply the foundation evenly – add water to water-based foundations or moisturizer to oil-based foundation if they become thick and difficult to apply.

3 Brush eyebrows in a neat line, pluck out stragglers if necessary, and apply water-based wand eye shadow in beige or peach all over the eye area from brow to socket, and *under* the eye around the cheekbones as a highlighter too. Blend in with cotton bud.

4 Apply shader with a rouge mop. Take up a brush full of powdered shader, shake off excess and press firmly into the natural hollow just under your cheekbones, blending upwards and downwards.

5 Pencil in brows with feathery strokes and a *sharp* eyebrow pencil (*don't* use an eye colour pencil – they are too soft for brows). Make a natural-looking arch, not too thin.

Even if you wake up feeling like nothing on earth, ten minutes will transform you into a very lovely lady!

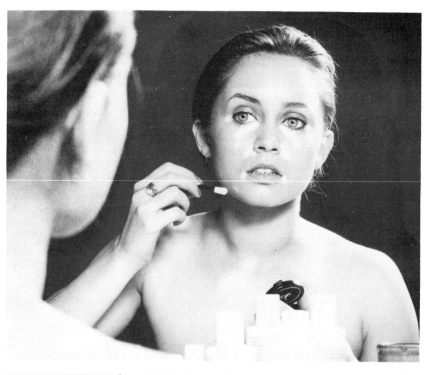

Covering those tell-tale blemishes with a light cover cream, applied after moisturizer but before foundation, will effectively even out your complexion.

Blusher is the best thing for making you look sparkly-eyed and healthy.

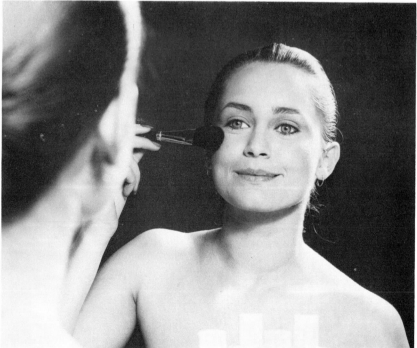

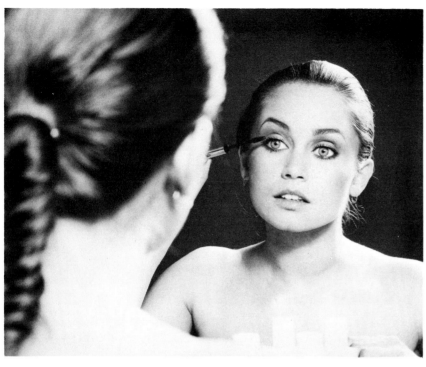

To avoid mascara splodges, stare wide-eyed at your reflection and stroke mascara wand upwards on upper lashes; look up slightly as you stroke downwards on lower lashes.

Bright lipstick is another instant reviver for jaded faces, but use a pencil first to outline your lips to prevent the lipstick 'bleeding' into the skin.

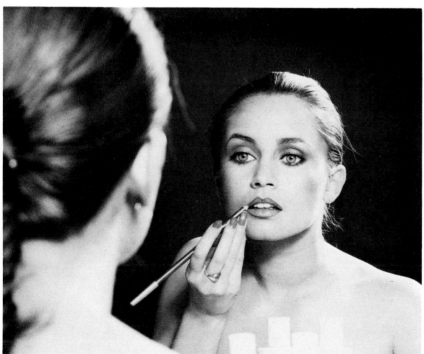

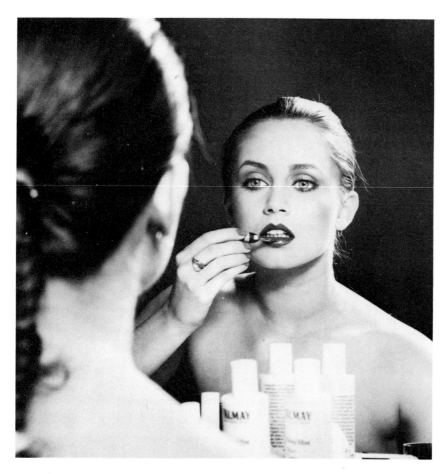

For a professional look, apply gloss over lipstick with a brush. Put it on the centre only of your bottom and top lips; it will spread out naturally.

6 Using a soft eye pencil in a darkish shade (brown or grey) pencil in around the socket area to the outer corner of the eye and down under the lower lid. Use the pencil *lightly* – if it's too hard, soften it in moisturizer on your hand. Now smudge the line with a cotton bud. This is the first time when shading tricks can correct eye problems: make your eyes look wider apart by concentrating on the *outer* lid, closer together by concentrating on the *inner* lid and bigger by concentrating on the centre of the lid area.

7 Now shade the lid itself, using colours to go with the clothes you intend to wear. *Suggestions*: pinky-peach on inside lid shading to deep plum on outside to go with brown or plum clothes; soft pearl grey shading to deep blue with jeans; cream shading to brown with a dash of gold in the centre with creams and browns; silver shading to gunmetal grey with evening blacks and shiny clothes.

8 You can use a kohl pencil in grey, brown or black (well-sharpened) to outline the lid and the inner rim of the lower lid.

9 Apply one coat of mascara to top and bottom lashes.

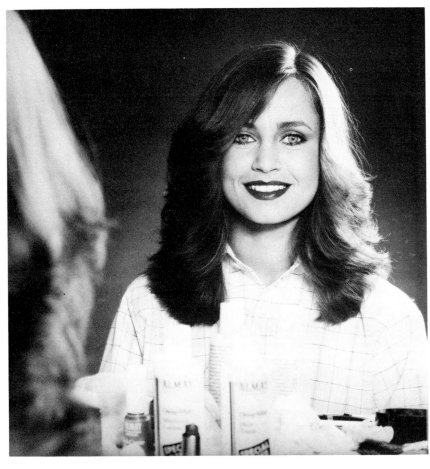

What a transformation! If you look terrific, you will feel terrific. *(Make-up: Almay; make-up artist: Patti Burris.)*

10 Pencil lip shape with brown or plummy (sharp) pencil, and fill in with lipstick. Top with gloss.
11 Apply a little extra blusher to cheeks.
12 Finish with an extra coat of mascara.

Sounds lengthy? The whole procedure really does take only ten minutes and it will last all day with extra lipstick and perhaps another coat of mascara later on.

The combined manicure and pedicure   *(32 minutes)*

You need nail polish and remover, orange sticks, emery board, cotton wool and cotton buds, hand cream. Place these items on a tray covered with an old towel. Remove socks, stockings or tights, roll up jeans, keep away from fluffy carpets.

1 Remove polish from toenails, then fingernails (toes are more tiring, especially if you're plump).

2 Remove grime and dry bits from behind nails and around cuticles with orange sticks, gently.

3 File into shape with emery board. Rub in hand cream (feet too!).

4 Apply polish remover again to nails to remove grease traces.

5 Separate toes with wads of cotton wool. Apply polish with three decisive strokes per nail, first the centre, then the two sides. Pause for a 30-second breather between each set of five. Your working order is: left foot, right foot, right hand, left hand. Remove odd blobs at once with cotton buds before they go hard.

6 Snatch a glance at the TV or have a drink; count to two hundred before applying a second coat.

7 Apply a second coat as above. A third coat won't be necessary if you use a rich, dark colour.

Shampoo and roller-set for medium-length hair

(35 minutes)

1 Plug in heated rollers – each roller should have a clean tissue around it to prevent tangling and to soak up any moisture left after blow-drying.

2 Assemble towel, shampoo and brush in the bathroom and plug in hair-dryer where you're going to do the job.

3 If you have a shower mixer attachment on the sink taps it will make the job much quicker. Strip top half.

4 Wet hair thoroughly, apply shampoo and rub well into scalp, allowing it to dribble down to the ends of your hair. Rub them gently.

5 Rinse thoroughly. Double washing is only necessary if your hair is *filthy*.

6 Apply conditioner to ends, comb through and leave for five minutes while you do facial exercises in the mirror. Rinse very thoroughly.

7 Wrap hair in towel, turban style, to soak up the drips.

8 Leave towel on head for five minutes (cuts drying time by more than that).

9 Dry hair with dryer and brush by an open window if it's sunny and warm.

10 Comb hair through and put in heated rollers. Make sure you take up small sections and hold them at right angles to your head. *Don't* let the ends kink when you're rolling up. Leave rollers in for about ten minutes. Remove, allow to cool, then comb or brush hair carefully. *Note* Wash-and-dry-naturally hair-dos are easy to dry rapidly under an angle-poise lamp while you do your nails, read or work.

18 Disguises for Disaster Areas

In the fifteenth century, make-up was used much more to *hide* facial problems than to embellish lovely features. In those days, pock-marks, scars, eczema rashes and scurvy spots were covered with egg-white or ceruse (a delicious brew of white lead and vinegar). These days, cosmetic disguise is subtler (much!) and cosmetic surgery is so sophisticated that no one need suffer from the really hideous kind of facial disfigurations that were common even fifty years ago.

But many people *do* have birthmarks and wonky noses, funny little piggy eyes, sticking-out ears and other disaster areas. Here's a guide to dealing with them:

Birthmarks and scars The 'port wine' kind of birthmark can be embarrassing when it's on the face or neck. Disguise is simple with a little practice. You need a special skin-masking cream (Innoxa's Keromask) in a tone slightly *darker* than your normal skin-tone. Apply it to the birthmark using a soft brush or your finger, blending the edges well. Now gradually lighten it with a white cream until you reach the normal shade. Then dust over with powder. A scar on the face can be treated in the same way. On the body, a deep scar can be 'filled' with a product used by theatrical make-up artists and a small palette knife and then disguised in the same way as the 'port wine' birthmarks.

Note Covering creams for camouflage are usually waterproof so they must be removed carefully with cleansing cream – not water. If you feel you need a lesson in the art of applying disguise make-up, your local hospital may be able to help. The British Red Cross run a 'beauty' service in many hospitals: find out the nearest one by contacting the Red Cross HQ, 9 Grosvenor Crescent, London sw1, enclosing a stamped addressed envelope.

Dark circles, bags and shadows Look to your diet – and your lifestyle – for the root cause of dark shadows on the face. Drinking more water and topping up the Vitamin C in your diet can often help. For instant disguise, invest in a small pot of cover-cream in a shade a little *lighter* than your normal skin tone, plus a fine brush. Apply your moisturizer as a base, then take up a very little cream on the brush and stroke gently over the dark area, blending in well. Allow to dry, then top with your normal foundation and powder. A light touch is essential.

Thread veins These usually occur on the cheeks, particularly when the skin is very dry and flaky in bad weather. Use a rich moisturizer and top the veins with a mixture of cover-cream and beige foundation – blend it in your hand and then use a brush to apply it. Don't use loose powder on top; instead press on a creamy compressed powder with a sponge. Sometimes these veins can be treated with sclerotherapy – an electrical method of dispersing the blood. See address on page 104.

Wonky noses If your nose is odd but not odd enough for surgery (and, frankly, I feel that surgery should *only* be contemplated if your conk is very embarrassing indeed) then try using make-up to help correct it. Dark shader applied to the tip of a long nose will help shorten it; applied to both sides of a flat nose, it will help make it narrower. Highlighter down the bridge of the nose will make it look narrow and aquiline. Plucking out the hairs between the brows can often make your nose look less pronounced (a good tip for men, too).

Piggy eyes Small eyes can be made to look *enormous* if you open up the eye area with pale beige or pinky-peach shadow all around the eye, topped with brown or grey shadow from the crease of the eye up to the brow and use kohl around the inner rim of the eye with lots of mascara.

Close-set and wide-apart eyes Darker shadows on the *outer* corner of the eyelid will make eyes appear wider apart; on the inner corner of the lid, it will make them appear closer together. The shadow can be part of your make-up – use softer colours with it and concentrate mascara on the outer or inner lashes to emphasize the effect.

Sticking-out ears Your hair style can cover your ears completely (both sexes!) and a soft beige foundation or cover-cream blended into the whole ear area can help make sure that when ears *do* show they don't look big, red and flappy!

Receding and double chins Check your profile in the mirror by holding a hand mirror at an angle. A receding chin can be helped with height on the crown and fullness at the back of your hair-do. A double chin can be disguised with highlighter on the tip of your *real* chin, shader blended in at the side and down over your neck. Don't sleep on high pillows and do 'lead with your chin'. Try clenching your teeth and pushing the corners of your mouth downwards to tone neck muscles. (But don't do it in public!)

Cosmetic surgery Despite regular letters from readers who write to me at *SHE* magazine asking to be put in touch with a reputable cosmetic surgeon, I'm afraid that I *can't* recommend one – either here or in the magazine. Frankly, your own GP is the best person to ask for initial advice and if he or she proves unhelpful, then your local hospital may be able to advise you. Do make sure that you have the fullest consultation with your surgeon before the 'op'. If he's at all sketchy during a pre-op discussion, opt out fast! The discussion should include what the results are likely to be and how much 'discomfort' (another word for pain) is involved. Clinics are springing up all over the place for this lucrative work and, while some of them are excellent, some most definitely are not.

Cosmetic surgery is pretty expensive, although it is available on the National Health if the problem is causing you acute embarrassment and your doctor recommends surgery. Expect to pay from £350 for a 'nose job'; from £300 for a face lift and eyelid operation; and from £750 for the more serious tummy, thigh and buttock lifts. Operations are also available combined with holidays abroad or in this country – but the holiday atmosphere is rather dampened by that droopy, post-operative feeling!

Here is a guide to the procedures used for various operations which are currently possible. Bosom surgery is discussed on page 50.

Face lift (rhytidoplasty) This helps remove wrinkles, loose skin and sagging folds. It won't remove deep forehead lines. The incision is made in front of the ears and the stitches do show, although they fade a little in time. The operation involves a stay of three to five days in the clinic, and the stitches are removed after ten days. The face is swollen and uncomfortable at first. Recommended only if your lines and bags are really unsightly and ruining your life! The recent transformation of Mrs Betty Ford, wife of ex-president Gerald Ford, certainly was dramatic, but she looked a lot healthier and more rested as well.

Nose remodelling (rhinoplasty) The most popular type of cosmetic surgery involving the re-structuring of bone and/or cartilage and flesh to remodel the nose. The surgeon usually prefers to work with a local anaesthetic only (tubes would interfere with the delicate work involved) which can be scary. Bruising and 'discomfort' occur and continue for several weeks. However, they are well worth suffering if you have an enormous or horribly badly-shaped nose.

Eyelid surgery (blepharoplasty) In addition to bags under the eyes, wrinkles and loose fat in the upper eyelids can be corrected by surgery, and wrinkling and crows' feet can be smoothed out. Although the stay in the clinic is usually only two days for these operations, you need to allow about three weeks for the eyes to look completely normal. The tiny scars are tucked into the natural folds round the eyes, so they really don't show at all.

Tummy, buttock and thigh surgery A 'tuck' in the tum to remove excess flab (after childbirth, for instance) is becoming a more popular operation these days. Even the navel can be repositioned to a higher spot afterwards. However, this is major surgery under a general anaesthetic and the patient may need several months to recover. The same goes for 'bottom lifts' and the trimming of 'riding breeches' on the sides of the thighs. Try exercises and diet first!

19 Top to Toe Beauty Guide

Take a long cool look at yourself. If you hate what you see, consult my list of problems and remedies!

Problem	Cause	What to do
Bosom		
Droopy	Post-natal muscular droop due to stretched tissue; unsupported large breasts; slouching.	Wear supporting bra and do this exercise: sit before a small suitcase/briefcase/typewriter; press sides of case with hands and hold for a count of six; relax. Keep shoulders back always.
Too small	Breast-feeding; nature; heredity.	Augmentation operation involves inserting silicone prosthesis. Padded bras can add an inch or two. Do the exercise above to make the little you've got perk up!
Too big	Natural shape; heredity; successive pregnancy weight-gaining syndrome.	Reduction surgery works but is expensive and complicated. Wear a well-made bra; lose weight; wear dark tops with pale trousers/skirts. At night, flaunt your assets with plunging necklines!
Bottom		
Droopy	Natural shape aggravated by sitting on squashy cushions all day.	Sit on a hard chair; contract bottom muscles and hold for a count of six; relax. Do this as often as possible. Wear full skirts, not jeans. Surgery is possible although costly.
Just fat	Overweight, aggravated by above.	Knock bottom against a wall to break up fatty tissue. Lose weight. Do this exercise: lie face down on your tum, hands by sides; raise left leg as high as possible; cross over right leg and lower to touch floor; raise again, then lower to starting position; repeat with other leg.

Problem	Cause	What to do
Calves		
Hairy	Hormone balance can make some girls hairier than others; menopause.	Waxing isn't as painful as you might think and lasts for about a month. Electrolysis is possible but costly. If you have other hormonal symptoms consult an endocrinologist.
Fat	Overweight; lack of exercise; fluid retention.	Lose weight. Take more exercise: skating, walking, football. Put your feet *up* at the end of the day.
Thread veins	Blood leakage between layers of skin (can appear on face too) – people with fine dry skin are particularly prone.	Sclerotherapy reduces veins to bruises and they will fade as normal bruises do.
Varicose veins	Carrying excess weight or pregnancy; high blood pressure.	Lose weight. Wear support hose. Painful veins can be stripped out surgically – consult your GP.
Chin		
Saggy	Overweight; sleeping on high pillows with chin on chest.	Lose weight. Sleep on a low pillow or without one. Do this exercise: close mouth; pull corners down hard; hold for a count of six; relax.
Eyes		
Too small	Nature being mean.	'Open up' eye area with light shadow on lid and under eye; use kohl all round eye and lots of mascara. If eyes are deep-set, diminish brow bone with deeper shadow.
Too close	Nature again.	Try not to squint. Shift emphasis to the outer corner of the eye with subtle wings of coloured shadow. Pluck straggly hairs between brows to avoid frowning look.
Protruding	Nature or over-active thyroid.	Watch diet – you need zinc. Put dark shadow on lids to give illusion of depth.
Puffy	Late nights, TV, careless use of eye creams.	Sleep longer. Watch less TV. Pat night creams on lightly; drink more water; use cold teabags or cucumber slices as eye compresses.

Problem	Cause	What to do 100
Feet		
Tired	Badly-fitting shoes; too-tight boots; jobs where foot-work is necessary all day.	Cool in water with cider vinegar added. Buy comfy shoes with wide toes and arch support if you have to stand a great deal.
Loose or in-growing toenails	Pressure on the matrix (growing bed) of nail from shoes or boots.	Wear open-toed or roomy shoes. See your chiropodist regularly. If nail drops off, treasure the next one – they take about six months to grow!
Hair		
Dry	Under-active sebaceous glands; over-washing with harsh shampoos; bad perming; seawater; over-use of hairdrying equipment.	Switch to a mild shampoo and use conditioner. Have ends trimmed. Add vegetable oils to your diet.
Greasy	Over-active sebaceous glands; fatty diet; over-brushing; conditioner not rinsed out properly.	Cut out fried foods. Wash frequently with mild shampoo; have a light perm if it suits you to dry up the grease.
Dandruff	General ill-health; stress; hormonal activity (you can get pre-menstrual dandruff); recent colouring or perming.	Use a mild medicated shampoo; keep brushes and combs clean. Take Vitamin B or yeast tablets. If trouble persists see a trichologist.
Split ends	Hair abuse – over-heated rollers, bad perming, etc. 'Old' hair (over one foot long and therefore two years old) is bound to be tired!	Cut off worst ends; use protein conditioner to help repair damaged hair shaft. Step up protein and iron in diet; take Vitamin B or yeast tablets.
Alopecia (baldness)	Stress; shock; coming off the Pill; post-natal body reaction.	Post-natal and post-Pill alopecia will usually clear naturally. Treat other kinds with scalp massage. Increase protein and iron in diet. Hair transplant or wig for bad cases.
Knees		
Fat	Fluid retention; overweight; air pressure.	Drink lots of water and eat diuretic foods like oranges and lemons. Put your feet up at the end of the day.

Problem	Cause	What to do
Nose Ugly shape	Nature or accident.	Cosmetic surgery now widely available. Use shader to disguise minor bumps and bulges.
Shoulders Round	Bad posture; poor positioning during working hours; carrying heavy loads.	Sit on a straight-backed chair with desk at elbow height at work. Keep back straight. Do arm swings (backwards) when shoulders feel tired. Carry shopping in two bags; try and take the weight on your legs *not* your back.
Spotty	Synthetic fabrics next to the skin preventing perspiration evaporation; puberty; long hair.	Wear cotton next to your skin. Wash spots with mild soap and water twice a day; use a spot-drying lotion.
Skin Acne/oiliness	Over-active sebaceous glands; hormonal activity.	Clean skin several times a day with mild soap to ensure grease is cleared. Disguise with matt make-up. Avoid fatty fried foods.
Dryness	Under-active sebaceous glands; ageing; lack of sufficient oestrogen.	Nourish with suitable creams, choosing those which trap moisture in the epidermis.
Birthmarks	*Strawberry marks* are caused by vein leakage into spongey-textured top skin; *brown patches* caused by irregularity in skin pigmentation from the sun, the Pill or ageing.	Disguise marks with make-up: beige foundation topped with powder. Brown patches may fade if you come off the Pill or do not go into intense sunlight.
Scars	Surgery or accident.	Cosmetic surgery or make-up as above.
Teeth Dingy	Persistent plaque; smoking; drinking lots of beer/wine; bad brushing.	Have a scale and polish at the dentist; use dental floss to clean between teeth; switch to a soft toothbrush with multiple tufts and *use* it.

Problem	Cause	What to do	102

Teeth

Crooked	Natural growth; compensatory collapse caused by teeth leaning towards a gap; diseased gums.	Orthodontic treatment: removal of tooth to give space to crowded ones or bridgework to fill the gap.

Thighs

Cellulite	(Recognized by French doctors as fluid trapped in subcutaneous tissue.) Lack of exercise; bad diet; bad circulation.	Go on fresh food diet; drink lots of water. Massage and pummel area with cream containing extract of ivy.
Mottled skin	Poor circulation; too-tight jeans; pressing legs against radiators.	Get blood circulating with exercise and massage. Fake or real tan will cover mottled marks.
Hairy	Dark hair growth becomes more intense with ageing.	Waxing is effective for about a month. Electrolysis removes hairs permanently but should be done in winter as scars take some time to heal.

Tummy

Flabby	Post-natal sag; lack of tummy muscle use; eating vast meals every night; constipation; overweight.	Eat small high-fibre meals more often. Swim, play tennis; hold tummy in when walking and sitting. Do this exercise: lie on the floor on your back, feet hooked under a heavy piece of furniture; sit up slowly without using your hands; repeat five times.
Stretch marks	Lack of sufficient zinc in diet during pregnancy; lack of lubrication; sudden spurt of growth during puberty.	Use cream containing Vitamin E which seems to help the scars. A tan will help cover marks.
Thick waistline	Driving; sedentary life; overweight; tight jeans pushing flesh up.	Lose weight. Don't wear skin-tight trousers. Do this exercise: stand with feet apart; swing body loosely forward from the waist; swing to the right then the left; straighten up slowly.

Problem	Cause	What to do	103
Underarms Excessively sweaty	Over-active apocrine glands; hormonal activity; nervous tension and rushing about.	Use an anti-perspirant; wash area daily with a solution of one dessertspoon vinegar to one cup water. Wear cotton, calm down, do yoga.	
Upper arms Flabby	Unused muscles; overweight.	Diet if necessary, and do this exercise: stand with your back to a wall, hands by your sides; press palms against wall; hold and push for a count of six; relax.	

Beauty Addresses

Below is a list of useful addresses. Manufacturers quoted are always ready to give advice about their products, and will obviously be interested to hear if you have any complaints. Hair manufacturers are also keen to advise you on their products; send the fullest details and a hair cutting with any disaster stories!

Although all addresses and telephone numbers are correct at time of going to press, I cannot be responsible for changes. Do check by telephone before visiting the beauty schools and salons mentioned.

Beauty salons

London

Adam & Eve Salons
(Cathiodermie treatments)
4 Eltham Road
London SE12
01–852 7591

Micheline Arcier
(Aromatherapy treatments)
4 Albert Gate Court
124 Knightsbridge
London SW1
01–589 3225

Elizabeth Arden Salon
20 New Bond Street
London W1
01–629 1200

The Beauty Clinic
118 Baker Street
London W1
01–935 3405

Cosmetics A La Carte
16 Motcomb Street
London SW1
01–235 0596

Katherine Corbett
(General beauty treatments
   including sclerotherapy for
   thread veins)
21 South Molton Street
London W1
01–493 5905

The Face Place
(Try different brands of cosmetics)
33 Cadogan Street
London SW3
01–589 9062
and
31 Connaught Street
London W2
01–723 6671

Hawkins Clinics
(Cathiodermie treatments; there
   are also branches out of
   London)
42 Beauchamp Place
London SW3
01–589 1853

Headlines Hair & Beauty Salon
33 Thurloe Street
London SW7
01–584 9900

Marietta Kavanagh
(Cellulite and other treatments
  including face toning)
4a William Street
London SW1
01–235 4106

London Institute of Beauty
  Culture
247 Tottenham Court Road
London W1
01–637 1633

Molton Brown
58 South Molton Street
London W1
01–493 6959

Danièle Ryman
(Aromatherapy treatments)
Park Lane Hotel
Piccadilly
London W1
01–499 6321

Tao Clinic
(Write or telephone for the address
  of your nearest branch)
153 Brompton Road
London SW3
01–589 4847

Out of London

Adam & Eve Salons
(Cathiodermie treatments)
69 London Road
Sevenoaks
Kent
Sevenoaks 51231

Eileen Brobbin
(Electrologist)
37 Warwick Gardens
Worthing
West Sussex
Worthing 38111

Fingertips Nail Studios
(Write for the names of branches
  elsewhere in Britain)
29 London Road
West Croydon
Surrey
01–680 1504

Jean Graham Salon
(General Beauty Treatments)
253 Woollton Road
Childwall
Liverpool L16
051–722 3752
and
66 Bold Street
Liverpool L1
051–709 8150

Beauty and hairdressing schools

Alan International Hairdressing
  School
54 Knightsbridge
London W1
01–235 3131

Barbara Daly Beauty School
4 Chelsea Manor Studios
Flood Street
London SW3
01–351 1955

Christine Shaw
11 Old Bond Street
London W1
01–629 3884

Eve Taylor
(Post Graduate aromatherapy and
  residential courses)
Adam & Eve Salon
4 Eltham Road
London SE12
01–852 7591

Innoxa
(Specialists in camouflage for
  scars, etc.)
66 Grosvenor Street
London W1
01–493 1144

Joan Price Face Place
(Make-up and training school)
33 Cadogan Street
London SW3
01–589 9062

London Institute of Beauty
  Culture
247 Tottenham Court Road
London W1
01–367 1133

Mavala International Manicure
  School
139a New Bond Street
London W1
01–629 6174

Molton Brown
Advanced School of Hairdressing
58 South Molton Street
London W1
01–493 6959

Morris Masterclass International
247 Tottenham Court Road
London W1
01–637 1633

Cosmetic manufacturers

Almay Hypo-Allergenic
  Cosmetics
PO Box 17
225 Bath Road
Slough
Buckinghamshire
Slough 23971

Elizabeth Arden
76 Grosvenor Street
London W1
01–629 8211

Beauty without Cruelty
(Cosmetics with no animal-based
    ingredients)
37 Avebury Avenue
Tonbridge, Kent
0732–365291

Charles of the Ritz
51 Charles Street
London W1
01–629 8371

Cheesebrough Ponds Ltd
Victoria Road
London NW10
01–965 6575

Christian Dior
46 Mount Street
London W1
01–493 1957

Clarins
Joan Collings
85 Pennine Drive
London NW2
01–458 2172

Clinique Laboratories Ltd
54 Grosvenor Street
London W1
01–499 9305

Culpepper Ltd
(Herbs and postal service; allow
    for postage and packing)
21 Bruton Street
London W1
01–499 2406

Cyclax Ltd
Vale Road
Camberley
Surrey
Camberley 62181

Max Factor Ltd
16 Old Bond Street
London W1
01–493 6720

Germaine Monteil
33 Old Bond Street
London W1
01–629 1378

Princess Galitzine
Perlier Ltd
207 High Street
Sutton
Surrey
01–661 1618

Guerlain Ltd
22 Aintree Road
Perivale
Middlesex
01–998 9423

Sally Hansen
Hook Rise South
Surbiton
Surrey
01–397 5200

Johnson's
Johnson & Johnson Ltd
Slough
Buckinghamshire
Slough 31234

Kitty Little (AS)
32 Great Hales Street
Market Drayton
Salop
Market Drayton 3258

Lancôme
14 Grosvenor Street
London W1
01–493 6811

Estée Lauder Cosmetics Ltd
71/72 Grosvenor Street
London W1
01–493 9271

Leichner
14 Porchester Place
London W2
01–723 2509

Mavala Laboratories Ltd
139a New Bond Street
London W1
01–629 6174

Maybelline
1–19 Penarth Street
London SE15
01–639 4363

Miner's Make-up Ltd
Hook Rise South
Surbiton
Surrey
01–397 5200

Nivea Toiletries Ltd
Hook Rise South
Surbiton
Surrey
01–397 5200

No. 7 and Seventeen Cosmetics
1 Harewood Place
London W1
01–408 2191

Orlane Cosmetics (UK) Ltd
125 High Holborn
London WC1
01–242 1162

Outdoor Girl
Girl Cosmetics Ltd
Hook Rise South
Surbiton
Surrey
01–397 5200

Mary Quant
Hook Rise South
Surbiton
Surrey
01–397 5200

Revlon International Corporation
86 Brook Street
London W1
01–629 7400

Rimmel International Ltd
17 Cavendish Square
London W1
01–637 1621

Helena Rubinstein
76 Oxford Street
London W1
01–636 4111

Tu
F. W. Woolworth Ltd
242 Marylebone Road
London NW1
01–262 1222

Universal Beauty Club Ltd
(Mail order)
45 Weymouth Street
London W1
01–487 4318

Vanda Beauty Councillor
(Direct sales cosmetics)
18 Upper Brook Street
Mayfair
London W1
01–493 7852

Vichy (UK) Ltd
1–11 Hay Hill
London W1
01–492 0265

Weleda of Switzerland
(Herbal cosmetics)
Ship Street
East Grinstead
East Sussex
East Grinstead 25933

Yardley of London Ltd
33 Old Bond Street
London W1
01–629 9341

Hair care advice

Clairol
Bristol Myers Ltd
South Ruislip
Middlesex
01–845 5541

Clynol Advisory Service
(Perming and conditioning advice;
   salon recommendation)
Harefield House
Maidenhead
Berkshire
Maidenhead 32839

French of London
French & Scott Ltd
717 North Circular Road
London NW2
01–450 7232

Henna (Hair Health) Ltd
5–7 Singer Street
London EC2
01–253 5418

Inecto
22 St Margaret's Road
London W7
01–579 1221

L'Oréal Products
Berkeley Square House
Berkeley Square
London W1
01–629 8240

Redken Laboratories
(Write for the name and address
   of your nearest Redken
   franchised salon)
1 Albemarle House
Albemarle Street
London W1
01–409 2634

Wella Hair Care Centre
Basingstoke
Hampshire
Basingstoke 20202

Champneys at Tring
Tring
Hertfordshire
Berkhamsted 73326

Medically-supervised dieting and exercising programme, especially suitable for men. Physiotherapy, yoga, lectures, relaxation classes, indoor and outdoor sports, luxury rooms.

Chevin Hall
Otley
West Yorkshire
Otley 2526

Moderately priced with balanced diets, beauty treatments. Their speciality is a five-day course.

Granny's Beautiful Bodies Ltd
2 Albert Gate Court
124 Knightsbridge
London SW1
01–581 1261

Classes include general exercise based on yoga, jazz, ballet directed by Jo Kemp, children's movement. Reasonable prices per lesson or per course.

Henlow Grange Health Farm
Hitchin
Hertfordshire
Hitchin 811111

Luxury facilities including pool, mud baths; beauty treatments, dieting.

Inglewood Health Hydro
Kingsbury
Berkshire
Hungerford 2022

Luxury stately home with facilities for osteopathy, electrotherapy, physiotherapy, massage, sauna, steam baths, hydro-therapy; medically supervised diets, beauty treatments.

Kilkea Castle
Castledermont
County Kildare
Ireland
Carlow 45156

Luxury castle with separate sections for men and women. Sauna, gymnasium, plunge pools; full range of beauty treatments and diets.

Ragdale Hall
Melton Mowbray
Leicestershire
Rotherby 831 and 411

Moderately priced health hydro with excellent diets (supervised by *Slimming Magazine* experts) and beauty treatments.

The Sanctuary
Floral Street
London WC2
01–836 6544

Club for women only with day membership including use of gymnasium, swimming pool, sauna, solarium. Dance classes and beauty treatments also available.

Shenley Lodge
Ridge Hill
Radlett
Hertfordshire
Potters Bar 42424/5

Moderately priced with diets, beauty treatments, exercises to music, hairdressing. They specialize in a long weekend session.

Shrublands Hall
Cadenham
Ipswich
Suffolk
Ipswich 830404

Medium price-range with full health and beauty facilities, authoritative dietary advice.

Stoby Castle
Peebleshire EH45 8NY
Scotland
Peebles 6249

Luxury castle just outside Edinburgh catering for a maximum of twenty-six guests each week. Resident dietician, full range of beauty treatments and hairdressing; yoga, reflexology, aromatherapy, spot reduction and massage.

Town and Country Health
  and Beauty Salon
2 Yeoman's Row
London SW3
01–584 7702

Full slimming and beauty course arranged according to your needs. (Beauty School too.)

Westside Health Centre
201–207 Kensington High Street
London W8
01–937 5386

Club with day membership including use of sauna, gymnasium, specialized dietary advice from a qualified nutritionist, group movement classes. Men and women catered for. Special rates for squash courts and swimming pool.

Professional bodies

Write to the head offices of the organizations listed below for the name and address of their local member or branch.

The Acupuncture Association
34 Alderney Street
London SW1
01–824 1012

British Biothetics Society
(Secretary: Mrs M. Pilkington)
2 Birkdale Drive
Bury
Lancashire
061–764 3021

Institute of Electrolysis
Lansdowne House
251 Seymour Grove
Manchester M1
061–881 5306

Hairdressers Federation
11 Goldington Road
Bedford
Bedford 60332

Institute of Trichologists
Hair & Scalp Hospital
228 Stockwell Road
London SW9
01–733 2056

Women's Health Concern
16 Seymour Street
London W1
01–486 8653

NB The author and publisher cannot be held responsible for any problem arising from contact with any one of the manufacturers, salons or health farms mentioned.